6/20/78

Gene —
Enjoyed working with you.
Best wishes for a long
and successful career. —

Neil Farrelly

SURGERY OF THE PANCREAS
a text and atlas

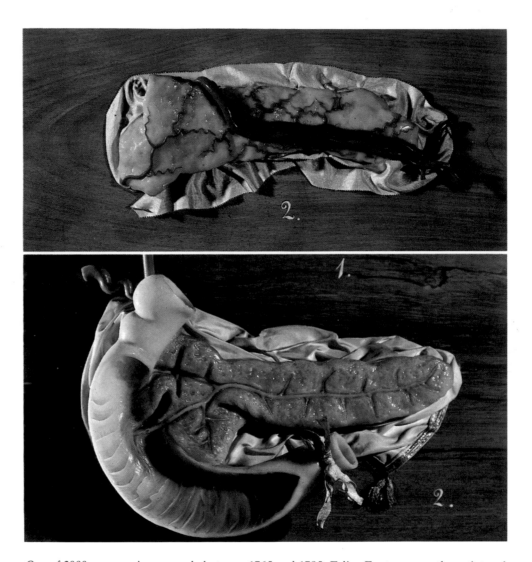

One of 2000 wax specimens made between 1765 and 1785. Felice Fontana was the artist and Paloa Mascagni the anatomist. This photograph is from the original untouched specimen (courtesy Prof. Erna Lesky, Chief of History, and Arthur Kline, M.D.). (From the Josefinum Wax Museum in Vienna, Austria.)

SURGERY OF THE PANCREAS
a text and atlas

Edited by

AVRAM M. COOPERMAN, M.D.

Department of General Surgery,
Cleveland Clinic, Cleveland, Ohio

STANLEY O. HOERR, M.D.

Chairman, Department of Surgery,
Fairview General Hospital;
Associate Emeritus Consultant,
Department of General Surgery,
Cleveland Clinic, Cleveland, Ohio

Original drawings by
ROBERT M. REED

Foreword by James T. Priestley, M.D.

with 273 illustrations

The C. V. Mosby Company

Saint Louis   1978

The C. V. Mosby Company
11830 Westline Industrial Drive, St. Louis, Missouri 63141

Library of Congress Cataloging in Publication Data

Main entry under title:

Surgery of the pancreas.

    Bibliography: p.
    Includes index.
    1. Pancreas—Surgery. I. Cooperman, Avram M.
II. Hoerr, Stanley O. [DNLM: 1. Pancreas—Surgery.
2. Pancreas—Surgery—Atlases. WI800 S961]
RD546.S953   617'.557   77-23621
ISBN 0-8016-1032-X

TS/U/B 9 8 7 6 5 4 3 2 1

CONTRIBUTORS

RALPH J. ALFIDI, M.D.

Head, Department of Hospital Radiology,
Cleveland Clinic

JOHN W. BRAASCH, M.D.

Chairman, Department of General Surgery,
Lahey Clinic Foundation,
Boston, Massachusetts

EDWARD L. BRADLEY, III, M.D.

Emory School of Medicine,
Atlanta, Georgia

SEBASTIAN A. COOK, M.D.

Department of Diagnostic Radiology,
Cleveland Clinic

AVRAM M. COOPERMAN, M.D.

Department of General Surgery,
Cleveland Clinic

GEORGE CRILE, Jr., M.D.

Clinical Emeritus Consultant,
Department of General Surgery,
Cleveland Clinic

CALDWELL B. ESSELSTYN, Jr., M.D.

Department of General Surgery,
Cleveland Clinic

LEOPOLD GONZALEZ, M.D.

Department of Diagnostic Radiology,
Cleveland Clinic

JOHN R. HAAGA, M.D.

Department of Diagnostic Radiology,
Cleveland Clinic

RUSSELL W. HARDY, Jr., M.D.

Department of Neurological Surgery,
Cleveland Clinic

THOMAS R. HAVRILLA, M.D.

Department of Diagnostic Radiology,
Cleveland Clinic

ROBERT E. HERMANN, M.D.

Head, Department of General Surgery,
Cleveland Clinic

STANLEY O. HOERR, M.D.

Chairman, Department of Surgery,
Fairview General Hospital;
Associate Emeritus Consultant,
Department of General Surgery,
Cleveland Clinic

STEPHEN A. KOLLINS, M.D.

Department of Diagnostic Radiology,
Cleveland Clinic

NORBERT E. REICH, D.O.

Department of Diagnostic Radiology,
Cleveland Clinic

EDWARD S. SADAR, M.D.

Department of Neurological Surgery,
Cleveland Clinic

MICHAEL V. SIVAK, Jr., M.D.

Department of Gastroenterology,
Cleveland Clinic

EZRA STEIGER, M.D.

Department of General Surgery,
Cleveland Clinic

To my loving wife, Jacquelyn, my children, Jeffrey, David, and Beth, who make it all so exciting and worthwhile, and my parents, Phillip and Lillian, who by example and love showed me how.

A. M. C.

To Janet, my loving wife and comrade of 45 years, and to our children and our grandchildren.

S. O. H.

I dedicate these illustrations to my wife and children, who through the years have shown me the patience, understanding, and encouragement so necessary to complete such an endeavor.

R. M. R.

FOREWORD

Any contribution to recognition and treatment of disorders or diseases of the pancreas is most welcome. This is especially true of *Surgery of the Pancreas: A Text and Atlas* by Cooperman and Hoerr. The text, which is lucid and concise, is based on extensive clinical and surgical experience, making it easy and instructive reading. Abundant references to the literature augment the authors' own experience. The beautiful and detailed drawings and illustrations by Robert Reed give pleasure to the eye in addition to furnishing technical help to the practicing surgeon. Chapters by colleagues of the principal authors concerning recently developed diagnostic procedures and selection of patients for surgical treatment are of great value and make this book far more than a surgical atlas. Presentation of divergent surgical views is refreshing and informative. The authors deserve appreciation for a significant work, which should be of value to all who are interested in the pancreas.

James T. Priestley, M.D.
Emeritus Staff,
Mayo Clinic,
Rochester, Minnesota

PREFACE

The pancreas has long been feared by surgeons as a dangerous, unpredictable, and treacherous organ. Any surgeon who has lost a patient to a fulminating acute pancreatitis after an apparently routine operation on a biliary tract or the stomach is unlikely to forget the experience. Cures of adenocarcinoma of the pancreas are a surgical rarity. The multitude of operations prescribed at one time or another for chronic pancreatitis testify to both the complexity of the problem and the lack of any comprehensive solution.

On the technical side, the proximity of the pancreas to the vital structures of the portal triad and the equally vital superior mesenteric vessels demands the utmost caution in operations in this area even when the anatomical relationships are not obscured by inflammation or tumor. Even biopsy of the pancreas should be regarded as a procedure to be done only for a clear and practical reason.

Surgery of the pancreas has been planned for the practicing clinical surgeon and surgical resident who may wish to review the techniques available for treating surgical problems which the pancreas may present. It is hoped that the illustrations and narration herein will be helpful. This volume also reviews the natural history of the diseases presented, the pathophysiology of some pancreatic disorders encountered by the surgeon, a discussion of the rationale of options open to him, and comments on the experience of members of the profession on the results of various treatments. The reader will note the frequent mention in these comments of the difficulty in evaluating clinical results because of the lack of prospective randomized studies and the complexity of factors affecting results.

Perhaps some of the readers of this text and atlas will help improve our surgical treatments by participating in carefully planned studies or by imaginatively adapting procedures to known pathophysiologic mechanisms or to knowledge still to come.

Our interest in pancreatic surgery has developed from the opportunities and teachings provided by our patients and colleagues. We are deeply indebted to these colleagues for broadening our knowledge and adding to our technical armamentarium.

The efforts of the many people who contributed to the publication of this text are gratefully acknowledged. We wish to especially thank Mr. Robert Reed, our collaborator and gifted illustrator, whose drawings are a testimony to his talent and industry; Rita Feran, head of the Department of Scientific Publications, who made good sense and better English of the text; Carrie Harris, Janine Willia, and Shirley Prokuski, who typed and retyped various versions (10^4); Renee Gutman, reference librarian, who traced the earlier reference material; Dr. George Crile, Jr., who kindly reviewed many of the manuscripts as well as contributed a chapter, making as always timely and wise suggestions; the Photography Department of the Cleveland Clinic, who reproduced all prints for this text; and, last but not least, our contributing colleagues, whose chapters we regard as both current and comprehensive.

Avram M. Cooperman
Stanley O. Hoerr

CONTENTS

SURGERY OF THE PANCREAS
a text and atlas

CHAPTER 1

Anatomy of surgical approaches and incisions for pancreatic surgery

AVRAM M. COOPERMAN
EZRA STEIGER

The pancreas is a retroperitoneal organ which has been divided (for convenience) into five portions: the head, neck, body, tail, and uncinate process (Fig. 1-1). There are no impressions on its external surface to delineate these divisions; but the superior mesenteric vessels, lying posteriorly, subdivide the gland into the head (that portion to the right of the vessels), neck (that portion lying over the vessels), and body and tail (that portion to the left of the vessels). The uncinate process lies posterior to the superior mesenteric vein.

The dimensions of the pancreas are variable, but the gland measures 15 to 20 cm in length and weighs 80 to 90 grams.

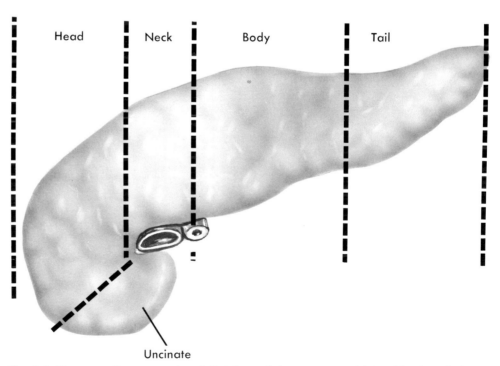

Fig. 1-1. There are five anatomic subdivisions of the pancreas which utilize its relation to the superior mesenteric vein and artery.

EMBRYOLOGY

The pancreas develops from two anlagen, a ventral and a dorsal (Fig. 1-2).

The ventral portion is formed by an outpouching from the bud which gives rise to the liver, gallbladder, and common duct. The duct drainage to this segment is through the duct of Wirsung. After the ventral segment rotates to the right and posterior to the duodenum, it forms the head of the pancreas and fuses with the dorsal segment to form the uncinate process.

The dorsal portion of the pancreas arises as a direct outpouching from the duodenum. It forms part of the uncinate process and the body and tail of the gland. Its drainage is via the duct of Santorini, which is usually of minor importance in adults.

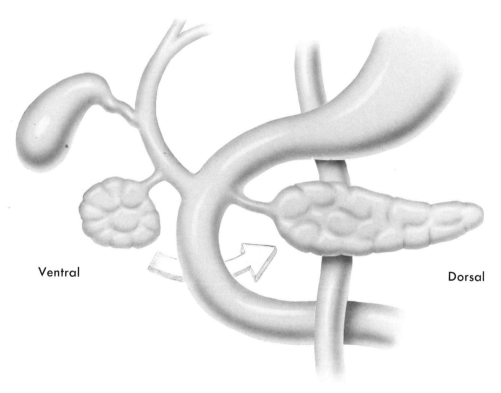

Ventral

Dorsal

Fig. 1-2. The pancreas is derived from a ventral and a dorsal bud. The ventral segment arises from the same bud as the gallbladder, liver, and common bile duct. The dorsal segment is a direct outpouching of the duodenum.

ARTERIAL SUPPLY

The major arterial supply to the pancreas is derived from the celiac axis and the superior mesenteric artery (Fig. 1-3).

Although inaccurate, it is simpler to think of two arterial divisions to the pancreas: one supplying the head and uncinate process, the other supplying the neck, body, and tail (Fig. 1-4). This inaccuracy (due to the ample collaterals between both arterial systems) serves to emphasize that the blood supply to the head comes primarily from branches of the gastroduodenal and superior mesenteric arteries whereas the supply to the neck, body, and tail comes from the splenic artery (Fig. 1-4).

The major arterial distribution to the head of the gland is from the anterior and posterior pancreaticoduodenal arteries. There are two divisions: a superior and an inferior. The superior vessels are branches of the gastroduodenal artery; the inferior vessels arise from the posterior surface of the superior mesenteric artery.

The splenic artery courses above and parallel with the neck, body, and tail of the pancreas. During this course multiple small branches are given off to the superior surface of the gland. The most important branches are the great pancreatic (pancreatica magna) and dorsal pancreatic arteries.

The dorsal pancreatic artery arises from the splenic artery one third of the time, and from the celiac axis another third. It courses through the pancreas toward the inferior surface, where at a varying distance from the edge it divides into a right and a left branch. The right branch supplies the head and uncinate process of the pancreas. The left branch (pancreatica inferior) supplies the body and tail of the gland. The left branch is constant and is found in 96% to 100% of dissected specimens.

VENOUS DRAINAGE

The venous drainage of the pancreas has not been studied as well as the arterial system. Whereas most branches follow the arteries, the venous tributaries eventually course to either the splenic or the superior mesenteric vein. They are numerous, short, and frequently a surgical nuisance.

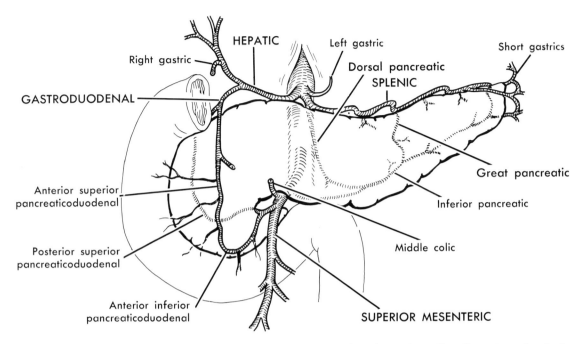

Fig. 1-3. The arterial supply to the pancreas arises from the celiac (hepatic and splenic arteries) and the superior mesenteric artery. The blood supply to the head of the gland is via the pancreaticoduodenal (anterior and posterior) arcades, which arise from the gastroduodenal artery (superior) and superior mesenteric arteries (inferior).

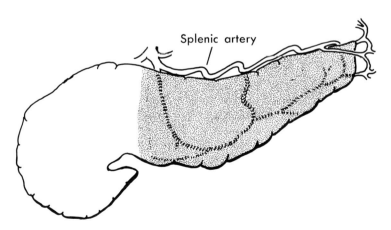

Fig. 1-4. The major arterial supply to the body and tail of the pancreas is derived from branches of the splenic artery.

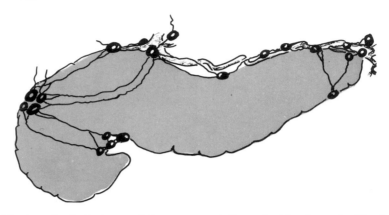

Fig. 1-5. The lymphatic drainage of the pancreas follows the blood supply. The lymphatics draining the body and tail enter the splenic hilar nodes. The lymphatics from the head and uncinate process drain along both arcades and then into the hepatic or mesenteric nodes.

LYMPHATICS

As shown in Fig. 1-5, the lymphatics of the pancreas drain into numerous channels and in multiple directions. Those draining the tail enter the splenic hilar nodes; those from the body and head enter the pancreaticoduodenal nodes (along both vascular arcades), where they may drain into the hepatic or left gastric nodes or into the nodes along the lower border of the pancreas and the superior mesenteric artery.

DUCTS

The origins of the ventral duct of Wirsung and the dorsal duct of Santorini have been explained. Though variations do occur, in 90% of patients there is a communication between the dorsal and ventral pancreatic duct systems (often seen on cholangiograms) (Fig. 1-6). These join the common duct and enter the duodenum through one opening.

The frontispiece of this book is a wax specimen made in the seventeenth century depicting the major duct drainage of the pancreas. There has been little added to our knowledge of the gland since that time. A recent technique to study pancreatic anatomy has been latex fixation of the pancreatic vessels and ducts with digestion of the acinar tissue. The myriads of ducts seen in Fig. 1-7 represent a small segment of duct drainage from normal acinar tissue. Although the duct of Santorini is of major importance for drainage in some patients, most anomalies are related to its position or the site of its opening into the duodenum.

INCISIONS (Fig. 1-8)

Any incision that gives exposure and access to the middle and left upper abdomen may be used for pancreatic surgery. Individual prefer-

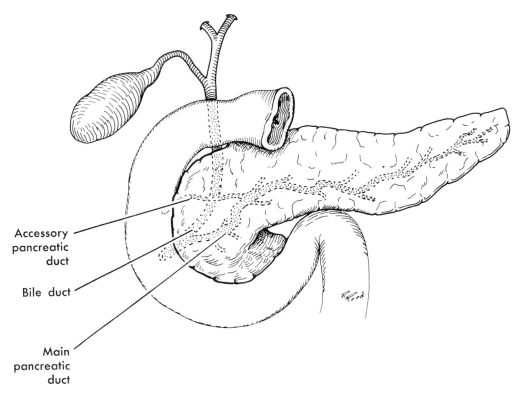

Accessory
pancreatic
duct

Bile duct

Main
pancreatic
duct

Fig. 1-6. The ductal drainage of the pancreas is via the main pancreatic duct (Wirsung) and the accessory pancreatic duct (Santorini). In nearly all patients the major drainage is via the duct of Wirsung. A single opening with the common duct exists in 90% of patients.

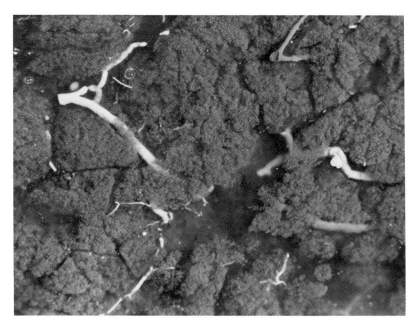

Fig. 1-7. Magnified view of a small segment of pancreas. The pancreatic duct has been injected and the glandular tissue digested. The myriads of tiny ducts resembling sponge are easily discerned. The white tubular structures are branches of the splenic vessels. (Courtesy Nick Stowe, Ph.D., Cleveland Clinic.)

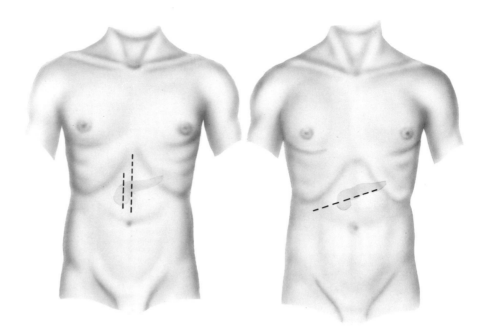

Fig. 1-8. Any incision that gives access to the upper abdomen may be utilized. Individual preferences will outweigh any suggestions. Our own bias has favored the upper midline incision. A right paramedian subcostal or oblique incision is used less frequently.

ences will outweigh any recommendations we might make. Though it is helpful to take into account the patient's body habitus, the angle of the costal arch, previous abdominal surgery, and the suspected location of the pathology—our own "habits" have generally favored an upper midline incision, extending from the xiphoid process to or below the umbilicus. In obese individuals or those with a wide costal arch, a right upper abdominal oblique incision carried to the opposite arch is used. We have infrequently used the bilateral subcostal incision favored by many surgeons. Also used infrequently but of value is a right subcostal or lateral extension off the midline incision.

EXPLORATION OF THE PANCREAS (Fig. 1-9)

After an incision has been made that is comfortable for the surgeon and gives access to the pancreas, a careful and thorough exploration of the peritoneal cavity is done. Satisfied with visual and/or manual inspection of all viscera, the surgeon is then ready to approach the pancreas.

There are, of course, many ways to explore the pancreas. *Any method that is thorough and provides satisfactory exposure of the gland may be used.*

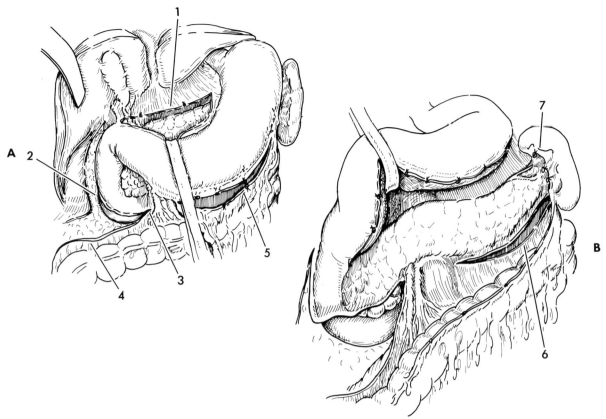

Fig. 1-9. Exploration of the pancreas. **A,** *1,* With traction on the stomach displacing it downward and to the left, the gastrohepatic omentum is incised lateral to the left gastric vein and the nerves of Latarjet. This allows visualization and palpation of the neck and body of the gland. *2* and *3,* The duodenum is next pulled to the left and the peritoneum over the descending duodenum incised. The dissection can be carried to the mesenteric vessels below and allows visualization of the inferior vena cava medially. *4,* If the patient is obese or exposure of the third portion of the duodenum incomplete, an important maneuver is to incise the peritoneum overlying the right and transverse colon and reflect the ascending and right transverse colon downward. Complete exposure of the third portion of the duodenum is thereby obtained. *5,* The gastrocolic omentum is next incised. This tissue plane is easier to enter toward the left, where the tissue is thinner and avascular and where the mesocolon and middle colic artery are less easily injured. The opening is widened and the stomach retracted upward by a malleable retractor or a drain placed around the stomach. This then allows complete visualization of the neck, body, and tail of the gland. **B,** *6,* The avascular plane of tissue beneath the inferior portion of the pancreas is incised to permit bimanual palpation of the gland. *7,* Finally, if it is difficult to develop a tissue plane beneath the pancreas because of inflammation or scarring, medial rotation of the spleen delivers the tail of the gland into a more accessible location. Planned splenectomy is generally unnecessary.

CLOSURE

As with incisions, the type and manner of closure will depend on individual preferences. Our recommendations include the use of nonabsorbable suture material for the fascial layers and the liberal use of drains after resections.

REFERENCES

1. Berman, L. G., Prior, J. T., Abramow, S. M., and Ziegler, D. D.: A study of the pancreatic duct in man by the use of vinyl acetate casts of postmortem preparations, Surg. Gynecol. Obstet. **110:**391, 1960.
2. Hollinshead, H.: Anatomy for surgeons. Vol. 2. The thorax, abdomen, and pelvis, New York, 1956, Harper & Bros.
3. White, T. T.: Surgical anatomy of the pancreas. In Carey, L. C., editor: The pancreas, St. Louis, 1973, The C. V. Mosby Co.

CHAPTER 2

Diagnostic procedures

Conventional roentgenographic diagnosis

STEPHEN A. KOLLINS

Roentgenographic diagnosis of pancreatic disease has been difficult for many reasons. The retroperitoneal location of the pancreas and the lack of correlation between roentgenographic and physical findings are two important factors. Optimal roentgenographic examination must be performed and interpretation skillfully accomplished, with pancreatic disease highly suspected if early diagnosis can be approached. Recent advances in computed tomography and ultrasound have provided two new dimensions in the diagnosis of pancreatic disease. Both techniques have led to a greater appreciation of the unique anatomic relationships of the pancreas; but they are not available in many institutions, where routine diagnostic procedures must be utilized.

Cooperation between the clinician and radiologist is essential, for often the roentgenographic findings must be interpreted when the symptoms are not specific. Unfortunately many of the plain film findings in the abdomen, chest, or extremities associated with pancreatic disease are also nonspecific; and occasionally extensive pancreatic disease is present with minimal roentgenographic changes.

Plain film examinations, barium studies of the upper gastrointestinal tract, and hypotonic duodenography are used to evaluate pancreatic disease. These procedures are relatively inexpensive and readily available. However, their diagnostic accuracy is limited by several factors:

    1. Changes in the viscera adjacent to the pancreas are nonspecific. Both inflammatory and neoplastic pancreatic processes can pro-

I thank Mortimer Lubert, M.D., Mount Sinai Hospital, Cleveland, for sharing case material, some of which is illustrated here.

duce similar duodenal changes. Similar abnormal findings may indicate primary duodenal disease or may be seen in normal individuals as a transient phenomenon.

2. Extensive malignancy of the body and tail of the pancreas may be present with neither clinical nor roentgenographic findings.

3. Examination of the duodenum may be difficult because of active duodenal peristalsis, which can occur normally or be heightened by adjacent inflammatory disease.

Hypotonic duodenography has helped considerably in evaluating the "difficult" duodenum which either is poorly seen at barium examination due to hypermotility or is suspiciously abnormal. When spasm or peristalsis is eliminated by pharmacologic paralysis of the duodenum, lesions can be more clearly demonstrated in multiple projections or with air contrast. Normal peristaltic activity mimicking either duodenal or periduodenal disease may be recognized, obviating further evaluation or even surgery. A tubeless examination[10,16] may supplement the conventional barium study, but in most instances an intubated hypotonic duodenogram provides the necessary information.

Hypotonic duodenography has been reviewed in two monographs.[5,12] Although intubated duodenography is clearly more accurate for evaluating the duodenum or pancreas than is the conventional barium meal,[5] the latter is more acceptable to the patient and may provide the required information. In our practice conventional barium examination is performed first and supplemented if necessary by duodenography. The increased use of computed tomography recently has minimized the need for duodenography.

ACUTE PANCREATITIS

Acute pancreatitis may vary in its clinical presentation,[9] and for many patients plain films of the abdomen and chest are the only roentgenographic studies performed because of the patient's precarious state of health. One should recognize that plain abdominal films may be normal in two third of patients with acute pancreatitis.[28] Other investigators, however, report abnormal findings with greater frequency.[5] These abdominal findings vary from patient to patient and depend on the severity and duration of the inflammatory process.

The most common abnormal finding in acute pancreatitis is dilatation of a loop of adjacent small bowel—the "sentinel loop" (Figs. 2-1 and 2-2). Although a nonspecific finding, it has been reported in as many as 55% of patients with acute pancreatitis.[27] It is usually located in the left upper quadrant but may be seen wherever a collection of inflammatory exudate irritates the adjacent bowel.

Usually the remaining small bowel contains little or no gas (Fig. 2-1), but occasionally the nonobstructive ileus is generalized as was observed in 12% of the patients with pancreatitis reported by Cantwell and Pollock.[4] The observation that the walls or folds in the sentinel loop are thickened due to the intramural edema elicited by the nearby inflammatory process may be helpful. Felson[7] described the "gasless" abdomen associated with pancreatitis. The sign refers to the virtual absence of gas in the small or large bowel, usually with a minimal amount of air in the stomach. A similar appearance may be found in cases of high intestinal obstruction.

Air can distend the duodenum in both acute cholecystitis and acute pancreatitis. Weens and Walker[28] reported this finding with equal fre-

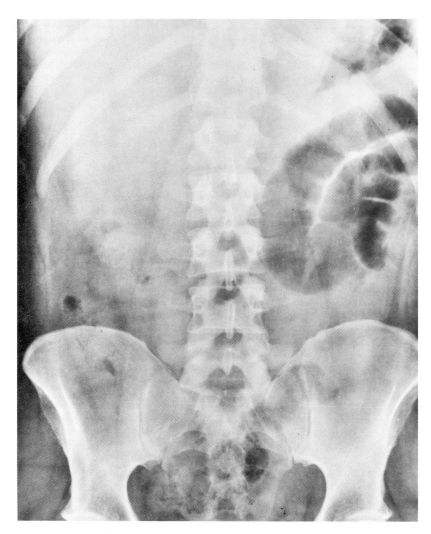

Fig. 2-1. Acute pancreatitis. Sentinel loop with an otherwise gasless abdomen in an alcoholic patient with delirium tremens.

quency in these two disorders, whereas Eaton and Ferrucci[5] found it more commonly in acute pancreatitis. This nonobstructive duodenal ileus associated with nearby inflammation is, in fact, a variation of the sentinel loop. When there is associated spasm of the distal duodenum, one may see a *duodenal cutoff* sign (Fig. 2-2). The air-filled duodenal loop may be deformed by the adjacent edematous pancreatic head, and thickening of the duodenal folds due to intramural edema may also be appreciable. Occasionally separation of the stomach from the duodenojejunal flexure and colon caused by marked edema of the body and tail of the pancreas or a collection of inflammatory exudate occurs (Fig. 2-3). Gastric displace-

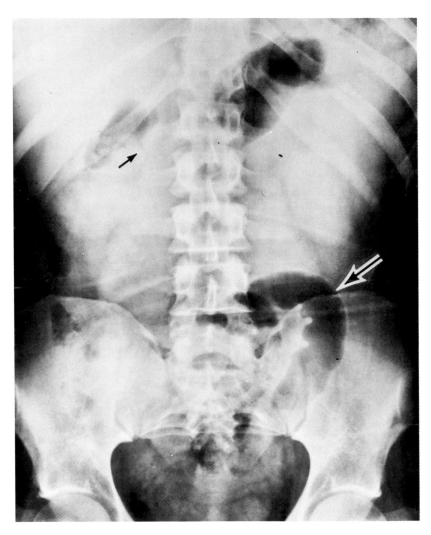

Fig. 2-2. Acute pancreatitis. Sentinel loop (large arrow) with a small amount of air in the duodenum. Narrowing of the descending duodenum (small arrow) is due to adjacent inflammation. Gas is present in the ascending colon but none distal to the hepatic flexure.

ment may also occur, but this is more frequent with pseudocyst formation or a pancreatic neoplasm.

The spread of pancreatic enzymes and purulent exudate along the fascial planes about the superior mesenteric vessels and transverse mesocolon may result in the *colon cutoff* sign: most often a gaseous distention of the ascending and transverse colon with little or no gas in the descending colon.[3] This finding is similar to that produced by obstruction of the splenic flexure due to a neoplasm, acute ischemia of the colon, or inflammatory bowel disease. Another colon cutoff sign may be distention of the ascending colon and hepatic flexure up to the right edge of the transverse mesocolon just to the left of the hepatic flexure, as has been described by Price.[20] Spasm in the transverse colon elicited by the adjacent inflammation may be the cause of the latter sign (Fig. 2-4). Neither colon cutoff sign is common, but either may lead to further study of the patient with a barium enema.

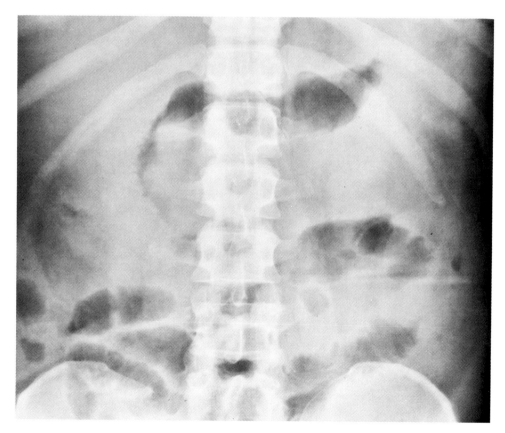

Fig. 2-3. Acute pancreatitis. Considerable air in the atonic duodenal loop, which is deformed by an edematous pancreatic head. The stomach is separated from the duodenojejunal flexure due to marked edema of the body and tail of the pancreas.

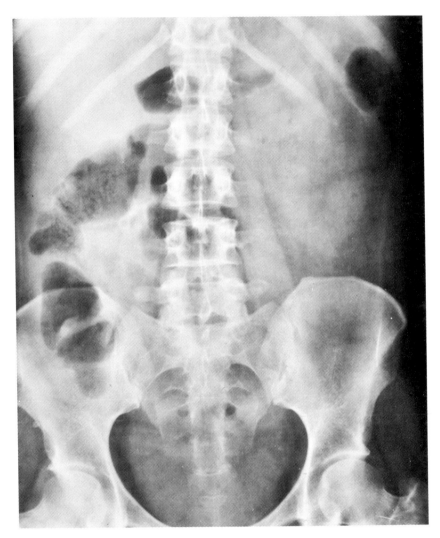

Fig. 2-4. Acute pancreatitis. Small amount of air in the duodenal bulb. Gaseous distention of the ascending colon and hepatic flexure with absence of gas in the transverse colon— the colon cutoff sign. There is a small amount of gas in the splenic flexure of the colon.

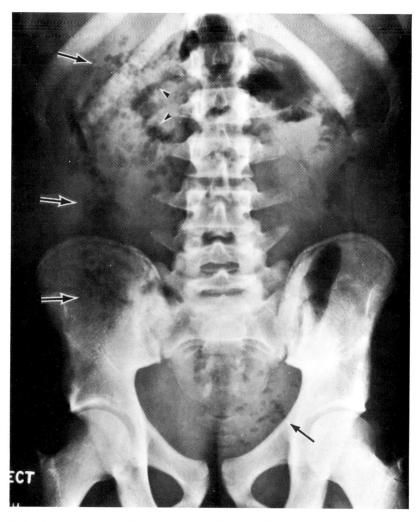

Fig. 2-5. Acute pancreatitic abscesses in an 18-year-old man. Pancreatic and retroperitoneal abscesses (bottom arrow) developed within 24 hours after he sustained blunt trauma to the abdomen. The inflammatory process dissected along the ascending colon with gas production evident (large arrows). The ruptured duodenum is deformed by adjacent edema (arrowheads).

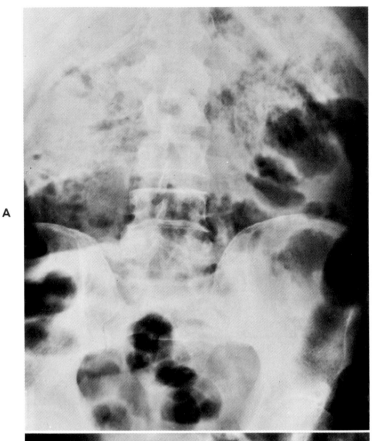

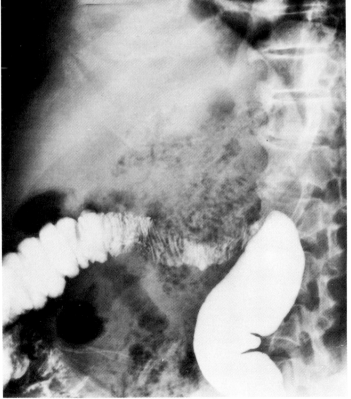

Fig. 2-6. A, Pancreatic abscess in an alcoholic adult. Extensive gas production in the retroperitoneum with changes in the right flank somewhat suggestive of fatty necrosis as well. Generalized colonic ileus. B, Inferior displacement by the abscess of the transverse colon and splenic flexure.

It is important to recognize that primary colonic disease can be simulated by the associated pancreatic process; the roentgenographic findings must be interpreted in light of clinical findings.

An abscess in and around the pancreas may develop as a complication of acute pancreatitis and portends a poor prognosis.[6] Early diagnosis is essential; even with surgical intervention, mortality is high.[5,9] Such abscesses may be seen as numerous bubbles of gas throughout the pancreatic region (Figs. 2-5 and 2-6). The gas may dissect along fascial planes and be seen paralleling the course of the colon. The abscess may involve the lesser peritoneal sac and in that case appear on upright or decubitus films as a large gas collection (Fig. 2-7) with or without a long solitary fluid level in the retrogastric region.

A mottled pattern of scattered ill-defined densities in the peripancreatic fat or retroperitoneum may result from the release of pancreatic enzymes into the soft tissues with subsequent hydrolysis and saponification of the fat.[2,14] The densities are almost pathognomonic of acute pancreatitis; but roentgenographic demonstration of this pattern is uncommon, in part because of suboptimal studies in acutely ill patients. Beren-

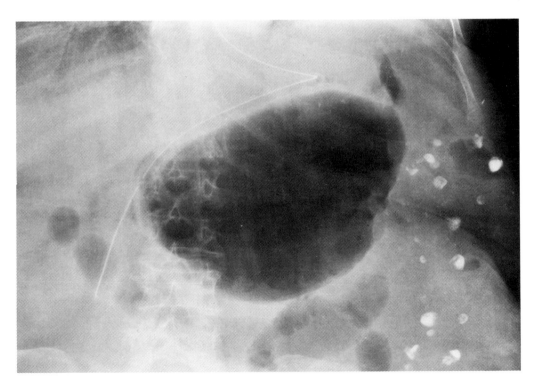

Fig. 2-7. Pancreatic abscess involving the lesser sac and complicating a perforated diverticulitis of the colon. The stomach is displaced anteriorly, superiorly, and medially by the large gas collection. The splenic flexure and transverse colon are displaced inferiorly.

son and co-workers[2] stressed that a high degree of suspicion is necessary for detection of this pattern but emphasized its reliability and prognostic importance.

The proximity of the pancreas to the diaphragm not uncommonly leads to intrathoracic changes in acute pancreatitis—including diaphragmatic elevation, discoid subsegmental atelectasis, basal nonatelectatic infiltrates, and pleural effusions.[8] The pleural effusions are more frequent on the left, though all these findings may occur bilaterally or on the right side alone (Fig. 2-8). These findings have been reported in up to 71% of patients with acute pancreatitis.[14]

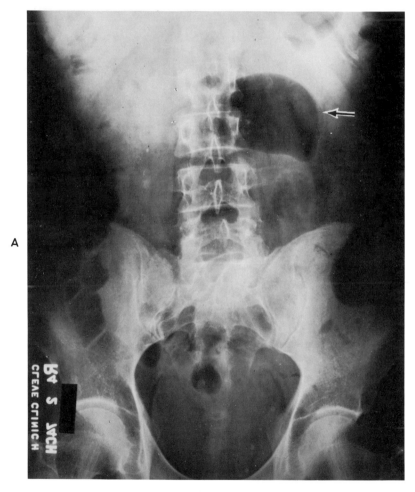

A

Fig. 2-8. A, Acute pancreatitis. Sentinel loop in the left upper quadrant (arrow). Scattered gas is present in the remaining small and large bowel. **B,** Pleuropulmonary abnormalities associated with acute pancreatitis. Left pleural effusion and left lower lobe retrocardiac infiltrate and atelectasis. Shallow inspiration is commonly associated with splinting of the upper abdominal muscles.

Although suppurative mediastinitis or abscess formation may occur with acute pancreatitis,[21] posterior mediastinal widening with documented pancreatitis also is suggestive of the uncommon extension of a pseudocyst through either the esophageal or the para-aortic hiatus into the chest. These inferior mediastinal masses usually are located in the retrocardiac region on the left, and most are associated with pleural effusion. Except perhaps for the rare mediastinal pseudocyst, all the changes in the chest are nonspecific. The presence of pleural effusion presents an ideal opportunity, however, for the ready confirmation of the diagnosis of pancreatitis. Determination of the amylase level in the pleural effusion readily distinguishes between the pleural effusions associated with pancreatitis and those associated with other intrathoracic or subdiaphragmatic inflammatory processes.

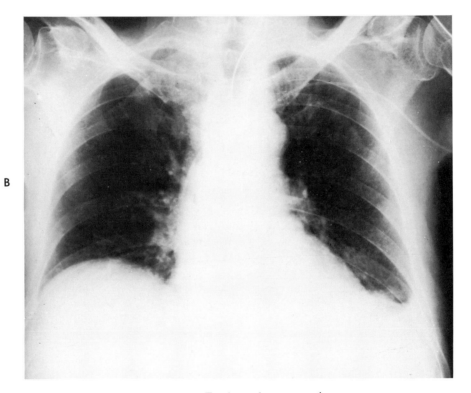

B

Fig. 2-8, cont'd. For legend see opposite page.

CHRONIC PANCREATITIS

Pancreatic calcification, though uncommonly reported in cases of acute pancreatitis, is characteristic of chronic pancreatitis. It occurs in about 30% of cases of chronic pancreatitis and is most often (75% to 95% of the time) due to chronic alcoholism. The calcifications may occur throughout the gland but are often of lobular distribution and more prominent in the head of the pancreas. When evident roentgenographically, they usually appear to be punctate and well circumscribed; they may also have a fine branching appearance (Fig. 2-9). Amorphous deposits in the fine radicles may have the appearance of diffuse parenchymal calcification, but this is less common.

The underlying process leading to pancreatic calcification has not yet been proved, but the calcific deposits which are often present within the ductal system most likely result from the precipitation of calcium carbonate.[18] Histologic deposition of calcium and lesions identical to those seen later during the course of chronic pancreatitis may be evident in biopsy material obtained before calcification is demonstrated roentgenographically.[22] This suggests that, because of its ability to detect more subtle

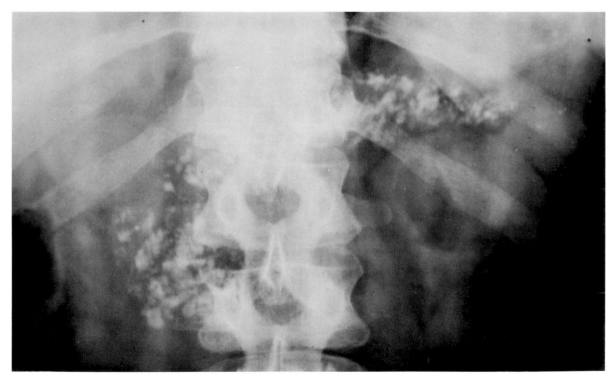

Fig. 2-9. Chronic pancreatitis. Typical diffuse involvement with pancreatic calcification.

differences in attenuation than is possible with film examinations, perhaps computed tomography will be of particular value in the early assessment of these patients.

Hereditary pancreatitis tends to produce larger and more rounded concretions than do other forms of pancreatitis (Fig. 2-10). The presence of calcification in members of a kindred known to be afflicted with hereditary pancreatitis is presumptive evidence of the disease even before symptoms develop[13]; calcification has been found in forty-two of nearly 700 members of twenty kindreds reported.[25] Familial hypoparathyroidism may also be associated with pancreatic calcifications, and the presence of both pancreatic lithiasis and nephrocalcinosis is highly suggestive of this possibility. Pancreatic calcifications in childhood suggest, furthermore, the concomitance of pancreatitis and cystic fibrosis. The latter disease, especially when severe and complicated by diabetes, is occasionally associated with pancreatic calcifications; but usually the underlying diagnosis is readily apparent well before the calcification appears. Malnutrition sometimes plays a role in the development of pancreatic calcification, but calcifications can occur unrelated to any of the foregoing factors.[22] Although calcification may occur with pancreatitis secondary to cholelithiasis, it is less common than with chronic alcoholic pancreatitis (Fig. 2-11).[5]

Calcification of the pancreas should be considered as evidence of a

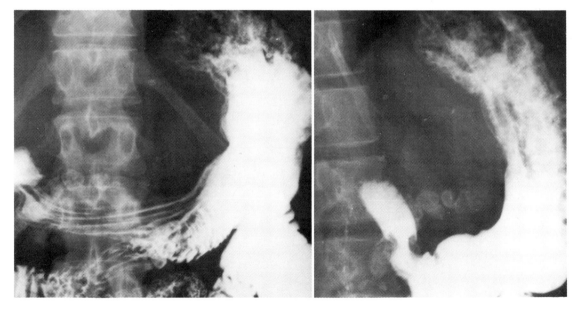

Fig. 2-10. Hereditary pancreatitis. The calculi are generally larger and more rounded or ovoid than with chronic alcoholic pancreatitis. Here they are oriented along the course of the major pancreatic duct.

benign pancreatic process. Nevertheless, there is a higher incidence of pancreatic carcinoma in patients with chronic pancreatitis, especially those patients with the hereditary form. The increased incidence reported varies up to 25%.[5] The development of pancreatic neoplasms or pseudocysts may be associated with either displacement or disappearance of pancreatic calculi, though calculi can also be passed into the duodenum. Calcifications have been reported in mucinous adenocarcinomas of the pancreas, malignant islet cell tumors, cystadenomas and cystadenocarcinomas, hemangiomas, and lymphomas. Malignant calcification is rare. A radial sunburst appearance with cystadenomas or calcified phleboliths with hemangiomas or lymphangiomas may provide diagnostic clues, but these are rare tumors.[18] Occasionally opacified stones in the gallbladder can be identified with pancreatic calcifications whether or not there are symptoms (Fig. 2-11).

Besides calcification in the pancreas, other plain film findings can suggest the possibility of chronic pancreatitis. Splenic vein obstruction with subsequent congestive splenomegaly may be due to either chronic pancreatitis or a pancreatic neoplasm. The splenic enlargement with inflammatory disease may be caused by thrombosis of the splenic vein as it courses along the upper edge of the pancreas or compression of the portal or splenic vein by a pancreatic pseudocyst. An enlarged gallbladder, seen as an ovoid soft tissue density in the right upper quadrant, is most suggestive of obstruction of the common bile duct due to a pancreatic or

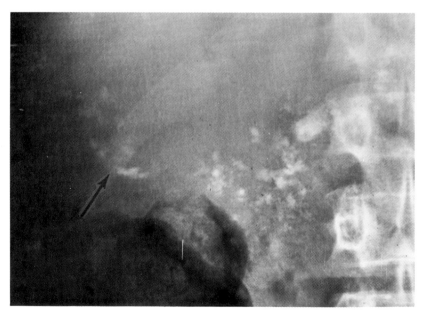

Fig. 2-11. Cholelithiasis (arrow) associated with chronic pancreatitis.

ampullary neoplasm. On rare occasion, chronic pancreatitis or even chole-docholithiasis can produce a palpable and roentgenographically demonstrable enlarged gallbladder. Ascites may be appreciated on a plain film of the abdomen and when due to underlying pancreatic disease is most likely caused by peritoneal spread of a neoplasm. Chronic pancreatic ascites, however, is being recognized with increasing frequency and may stem from peripancreatic lymphatic obstruction or leakage of a chronic pancreatic pseudocyst into the peritoneal cavity.[23]

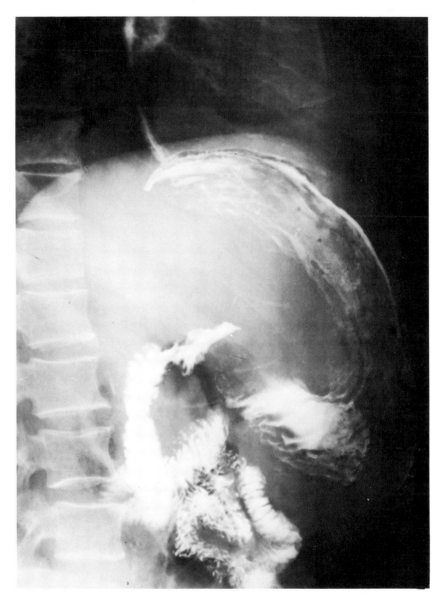

Fig. 2-12. Chronic pancreatitis. Marked anterior displacement of the stomach by a large retrogastric pseudocyst.

Other roentgenographic findings associated with chronic pancreatitis are related to pancreatic pseudocysts. These pseudocysts may develop within 7 to 10 days after acute pancreatitis. They are usually located in the region of the lesser sac and extend inferiorly and anteriorly between the stomach and the pancreas. They may occur, however, anywhere within the abdomen or pelvis. An ill-defined soft tissue epigastric mass is the most common finding on plain films, but pseudocysts may extend a great distance from the region of the pancreas (Fig. 2-12). Displacement of the

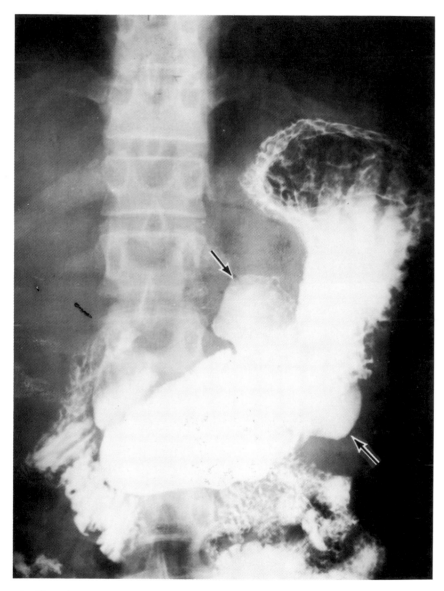

Fig. 2-13. Chronic pancreatitis. Upper gastrointestinal series demonstrating barium filling a retrogastric pseudocyst (arrows) after cystogastrostomy. For unknown reasons the cyst can be demonstrated only rarely in this fashion.

stomach and adjacent loops of bowel can be appreciated on a plain film, but usually upper gastrointestinal examinations are performed for confirmation. When arising from the head of the pancreas, the pseudocyst will often widen the duodenal sweep and displace the antral portion of the stomach upward. Pseudocysts arising from the body of the pancreas may displace the stomach upward or laterally if they extend around the lesser curvature. Pseudocysts in the tail of the pancreas displace the stomach anteriorly and usually medially (Fig. 2-12).[29] Because of the proximity of the pancreas to the upper pole of either kidney, pancreatic pseudocysts may simulate an avascular renal mass.[11] A pseudocyst of substantial proportions or strategically located may compress or obstruct the common bile duct and produce obstructive jaundice. Displacement of the colon by a pseudocyst can be appreciated on plain films, and a barium enema examination usually demonstrates an extrinsic mass displacing the splenic flexure and transverse colon inferiorly (Fig. 2-6, *B*).

Some pseudocysts resolve spontaneously, or they spontaneously drain into the gastrointestinal tract. Air or barium may rarely be seen within their confines after natural or surgically induced drainage (Fig. 2-13).

It is difficult to distinguish by barium examination between pancreatic pseudocysts and pancreatic tumors since pancreatic neoplasms may also indent the wall of the stomach extrinsically. Similarly a rapidly developing pseudocyst after an episode of acute pancreatitis may be associated with an inflammatory response sufficient to create an edematous, irregular, or even ulcerated appearance of the gastric wall. Approximately 80% to 90% of pancreatic pseudocysts are localized and diagnosed, however, on the basis of a conventional barium examination.[5] Computed tomography and ultrasound examinations may contribute to the diagnostic accuracy and provide additional means of following patients with pancreatic pseudocysts and assessing the natural history.

PANCREATIC NEOPLASMS

The roentgenographic signs suggestive of a pancreatic neoplasm vary with the site of origin of the tumor. Carcinoma of the distal body and tail of the pancreas constitutes approximately 25% of pancreatic tumors. These neoplasms are often large before clinical symptoms become apparent; they usually produce extrinsic indentation of the stomach, distal duodenum, and colon. Although these tumors are generally identified as extrinsic masses, there may be actual invasion of the wall of any of the adjacent viscera. In a retrospective series conducted on forty-six patients with carcinoma of the body and tail of the pancreas, changes in the stomach were observed in 83% and changes involving the duodenum in 76%.[15] Assessment of the retrogastric space by supine translateral[24] or axial pancreatic[26] views may aid in recognition of tumors in the body and

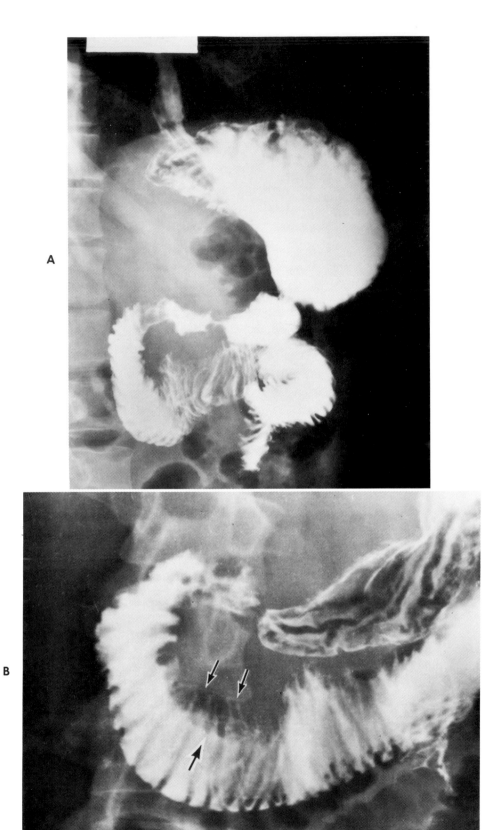

Fig. 2-14. Acute pancreatitis. **A,** Minimal deformity of the duodenal mucosa along the inner aspect of the third portion of the duodenum with a spiculated appearance. **B,** Similar spiculation of the duodenal mucosa in a patient with carcinoma (upper arrows). Note the suggestion of a double contour (lower arrow) due to partial indentation of the duodenal loop by an adjacent mass. The overall size of the duodenal loop is not increased.

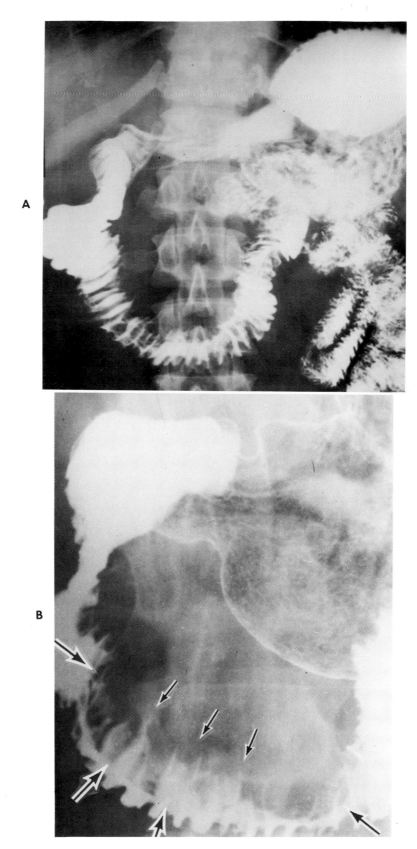

Fig. 2-15. A, Widening of the duodenal loop with spiculation of the mucosa along the inner aspect of the duodenum associated with pancreatic cancer. **B,** Spot film at fluoroscopy demonstrating more clearly the duodenal spiculation (small arrows) and double contour (large arrows).

tail of the pancreas; but regardless of the view, the most reliable evidence of the presence of a mass is impression on either the posterior gastric wall or the duodenum near the duodenojejunal flexure.

Carcinomas of the head of the pancreas occur three times more frequently than do those of the body or tail. Roentgenographic abnormalities are caused primarily by pressure of the neoplasm on adjacent mucosal surfaces or by associated edema or infiltration.

Deformity of the adjacent mucosa by a proximal mass or invasion of the wall by the neoplasm produces many signs that have been well described.[5]

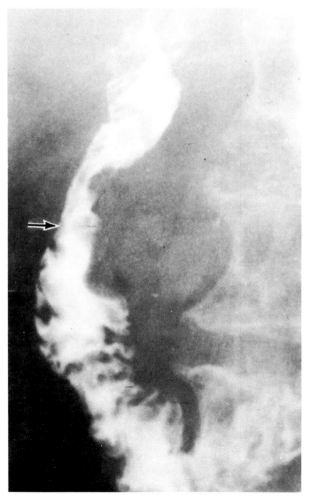

Fig. 2-16. Pancreatic carcinoma. Frostberg's "inverted 3 sign" is nonspecific and indicates an expanding mass in the head of the pancreas. Fold deformity probably is related to edema of the duodenal wall associated with the pancreatic neoplasm. There is either prominent edema of a fold or a tumor nodule in the center of the area of involvement (arrow).

1. The earliest sign is deformity of the mucosa on the inner curve of the duodenum. This deformity may result in a spiculated or brush-like appearance of the mucosa (Fig. 2-14) and is probably due to edema.
2. A small extrinsic mass may flatten the mucosal folds along the inner curve of the duodenum or may deform a coincidental duodenal diverticulum. Such straightening of the duodenal loop should not be confused with the normal straight segment below the promontory.

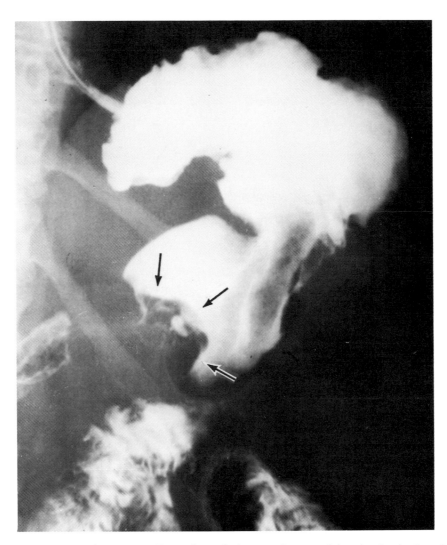

Fig. 2-17. Pancreatic cancer. Extension of the neoplasm, arising in the body of the pancreas, superiorly to involve the body and antral regions of the stomach. The neoplasm has infiltrated the gastric wall and produced a large central ulceration (arrows). Roentgenographically it appears to be a primary gastric carcinoma. The duodenum appears normal.

A slightly larger mass, which deforms a greater portion of the duodenal circumference, may produce a double contour (Figs. 2-14, *B*, and 2-15).

3. Further irregular growth of a neoplasm will sometimes produce a distinctly nodular appearance on the duodenal curvature. Continued enlargement of the pancreas may result in widening of the duodenal loop or actual displacement of the loop if the mass extends posterior to the duodenum. These last signs are also seen with benign inflammatory diseases of the pancreas and must be evaluated in light of

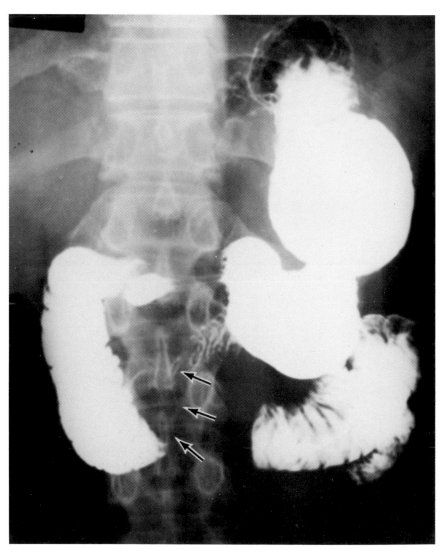

Fig. 2-18. Pancreatic cancer. The third portion of the duodenum is involved with a circumferential tumor mass which has caused obstruction with dilatation of the more proximal duodenum (arrows). Only a small channel through the tumor could be filled.

the clinical findings. Separation of the duodenojejunal flexure from the stomach may be produced by either a neoplasm arising in the body of the pancreas or an inflammatory mass. Caution must be exercised here, however, for there is great variation in the position and configuration of the normal duodenal loop.

4. The *inverted 3 sign of Frostberg* is also nonspecific and is probably more common with inflammatory diseases than with neoplasms (Fig. 2-16). It has been reported in up to 10% of cases of pancreatic cancer. Eaton and Ferrucci[5] attributed this sign to smooth muscle spasm and edema in the duodenal wall whether caused by a neoplasm or by inflammation.

5. Pancreatic tumors may extend through the adjacent stomach wall and produce ulceration mimicking a primary gastric tumor (Fig. 2-17), or they may encircle the adjacent duodenum and appear as an annular partially obstructive duodenal carcinoma (Fig. 2-18).

Ulcerogenic functioning islet cell tumors of the pancreas may also be suspected at upper gastrointestinal examination.[19] The indirect changes these tumors produce reflect the response of the antral mucosa to the secretion of gastrin by the tumors. The presence of ulceration, particularly in unusual or multiple locations, should alert the radiologist to this possibility. An excessive amount of secretions which may dilute the barium and interfere with coating of the stomach and small intestine may also demonstrate dilatation and edema of the folds due to excessive acid secretion. Other functioning islet cell neoplasms are not diagnosed by gastrointestinal examinations but may be demonstrated by angiography.[5]

It should be stressed that inflammatory and neoplastic enlargements of the pancreas often cannot be distinguished from each other. When direct invasion of the duodenum or stomach occurs, the infiltrative and destructive nature of the process may be apparent; but very often the roentgenographic findings demonstrate only the location of a mass in the pancreatic region. Findings at both plain film and barium upper gastrointestinal examinations may be nonspecific and indirect. The information gathered, however, when combined with the clinical history and physical examination often will accurately predict the location and nature of the pancreatic disease.

Endoscopic retrograde cholangiopancreatography

MICHAEL V. SIVAK, Jr.

The clinical application of operative pancreatography was demonstrated initially by Doubilet and co-workers.[34] Less invasive methods of pancreatography have been described,[41] but endoscopic retrograde pancreatography (ERP) is the most satisfactory. McCune and co-workers[38] performed the first endoscopically controlled pancreatogram, their work being followed by that of Oi[40] and others. A multitude of reports now emphasize the utility of endoscopic retrograde pancreatography and cholangiography.

The technique requires visualization of the papilla of Vater by a side viewing fiberscope in a sedated patient, followed by insertion of a catheter through the instrument and into the ampulla. A retrograde hand injection of a water-soluble contrast agent is performed under fluoroscopic control and roentgenograms are obtained. Because of its perpendicular relation to the duodenum, the pancreatic duct often fills first, requiring 4 to 5 ml of contrast agent. If the pancreatic and common bile ducts have joined to form one channel, both systems can be opacified simultaneously. In some instances important information is obtained prior to, or without, cannulation (e.g., pancreatic carcinoma invading the duodenum, primary carcinoma of the papilla itself). The pancreatic duct normally empties within 1 or 2 minutes, though a longer time period may be necessary in older patients; 20 to 30 minutes can be required for clearance of contrast agent from the biliary system. Success rates of 80% to 90% for opacification of the appropriate duct system can be realized with adequate experience.

Embryologically the pancreatic duct system arises from ventral and dorsal anlagen which shift to a position medial to the duodenum and fuse about the seventh week of gestation. In adults the main pancreatic duct (MPD) in the head of the pancreas derives from the duct of the ventral anlage, whereas the duct for the body and tail derives from the dorsal anlage. (See Chapter 1.)

There is often sharp angulation of the MPD in adults, sometimes with slight narrowing of caliber at the point of embryonic fusion. The proximal portion of the duct of the dorsal anlage regularly persists as the accessory pancreatic duct (APD), which in some cases communicates with the MPD. Although the APD is frequently visualized by ERP, it is patent and of caliber suitable for a secretory pathway in only a few cases. Cannulation of the APD can be accomplished in those rare instances when the primary route of the secretion is through the APD. Then the duct of the ventral anlage found in association with the common bile duct at the major papilla is rudimentary.

Roentgenographically the MPD is usually located within the span of the second to fourth lumbar vertebrae. It can narrow abruptly in its papillary portion and give the appearance of ductal dilatation proximal to the papilla. It tapers gradually from proximal to distal, though minor variations of caliber from point to point are encountered. The diameter and length of the MPD have been calculated in a number of autopsy, roentgenographic, and endoscopic studies; but because of differences in technique, the values are not strictly comparable. The approximate average length on the roentgenogram (corrected for technical magnification) is 15 cm; the normal range is wide, being 9 to 24 cm[43]; the mean diameter in the head, body, and tail is about 3, 2, and 1 mm respectively (corrected for magnification)[43]; but there is a wide normal range, so diameters up to 6 mm may be normal.

The branches of the main pancreatic duct (MPDBs) join the MPD in the body and tail at right angles, usually alternating with a branch from the opposite side (Fig. 2-19). This regular arrangement of the MPDBs is not present in the head. A large inferior unpaired MPDB which drains the caudate lobe of the pancreas is found in about half the cases.

The anatomy of the pancreas displayed by the pancreatogram is only that of the ductal system; the larger bulk of the parenchyma is not ordinarily visualized. The course of the MPD across the abdomen is quite

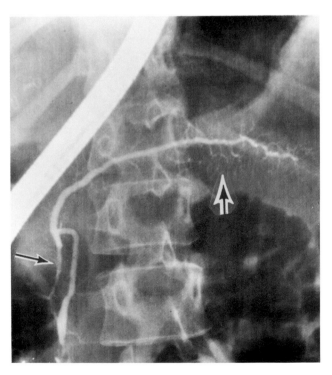

Fig. 2-19. Normal retrograde pancreatogram showing the accessory pancreatic duct (small arrow) and main pancreatic duct branches (large arrow).

variable, so interpretations of pathologic displacement are usually unreliable. The diagnosis of pancreatic carcinoma is therefore based primarily on abnormalities of the ductal system. Rarely defects in the filling of the MPDBs in a given area will suggest the presence of a lesion. The most common abnormal findings thus are obstruction of the MPD or a localized stenosis of varying length.

The sharply demarcated terminus of the MPD due to obstruction by a neoplasm is not hard to appreciate in the head of the pancreas. Obstruction in the distal body or tail can be more difficult to recognize because of the wide range of normal for duct length. Such blockage can be mimicked by inadequate filling of the MPD, but this source of error is decreased if the MPDBs are also observed to be opacified on the roentgenogram. Blockage of the duct close to the papilla may make retrograde injection impossible. Similarly obstruction can be caused by metastasis from other primary sites to the pancreas or by involvement with lymphoma.

Not every case of obstruction is caused by a neoplasm; shortening of the duct can likewise be seen with chronic pancreatitis or a pancreatic stone. Generally other changes in the MPD will suggest these diagnoses, but it must also be noted that chronic pancreatitis and carcinoma can coexist in the pancreas. It is possible to collect pancreatic juice for cytologic examination and thus further refine the accuracy of diagnosis.[36]

A high incidence of lesions in patients with recurrent acute pancreatitis will be found by ERP. Many of these will be surgically correctable, the operative plan often being based on the ERP findings.[33] Included among these lesions are common bile duct calculi, localized areas of chronic pancreatitis, and ductal obstructions such as calculi, carcinoma, benign tumors, and strictures (Fig. 2-20).

Early in the course of chronic pancreatitis, the ductal system can appear normal even in the presence of biochemical and clinical evidence for chronic pancreatitis. The earliest changes in the pancreatogram are found in the MPDBs. They become decreased in number whereas those remaining are shortened, dilated, and irregular. These findings are also noted with increasing age of the patient, so a diagnosis must be made with caution in older persons. In advanced chronic pancreatitis generalized dilatation, irregularity, and shortening of the MPD can be seen along with areas of stenosis and occasionally calculi within the duct (Fig. 2-21). At this stage the pancreatogram is diagnostic of chronic pancreatitis and there is good correlation between it and intraoperative observations, histologic findings,[35] and pancreatic function tests.[39]

Pseudocysts may be diagnosed by pancreatography, usually by filling with contrast when in continuity with the MPD or less often by displacement of the MPD or its branches. A tumor can also cavitate as a result of

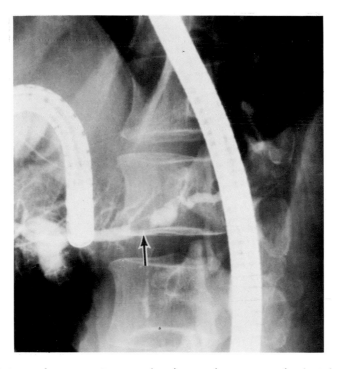

Fig. 2-20. Retrograde pancreatogram showing an intrapancreatic ductal filling defect. Cystadenoma of the pancreatic duct (arrow).

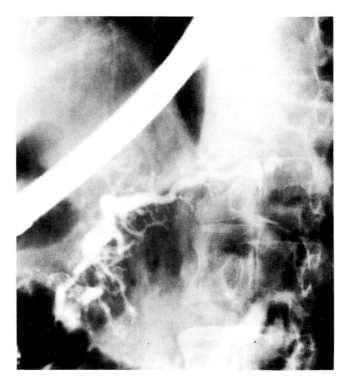

Fig. 2-21. Retrograde pancreatogram showing irregular dilatation, beading, and shortening of the pancreatic duct. This is characteristic of chronic pancreatitis.

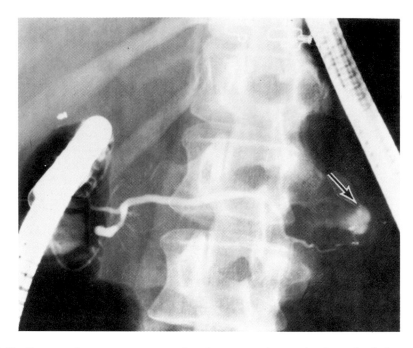

Fig. 2-22. Retrograde pancreatogram showing a pseudocyst in the tail of the pancreas (arrow).

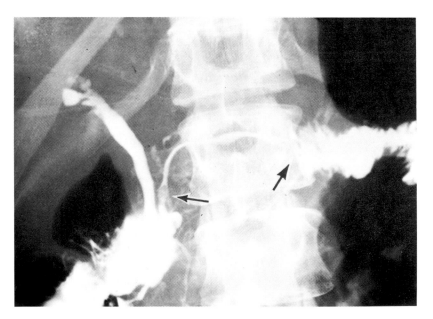

Fig. 2-23. Retrograde pancreatogram after a DuVal procedure (large arrow) showing an intrapancreatic ductal filling defect (small arrow).

necrosis; but these spaces will usually appear smaller, more irregular, and less circumscribed (Fig. 2-22).

The main complications of endoscopic retrograde pancreatography and cholangiography are sepsis and acute pancreatitis, each having an incidence of approximately 1%.[30] A minimum 2-week quiescent period during which the amylase value remains normal is recommended before the procedure. Hyperamylasemia, sometimes severe, frequently follows the retrograde study; but in most cases it is associated with no symptoms or sequelae. Sepsis occurs when there is filling of the common bile duct above the level of obstruction and with overfilling of a pseudocyst, which can be converted into a pancreatic abscess (Fig. 2-22). Early operative intervention is advocated in these circumstances.

Endoscopic retrograde cholangiopancreatography provides a special advantage for the surgeon preoperatively by defining the exact locations and nature of pancreaticobiliary pathology and by indicating those patients likely to be helped by surgery.[31,37,42,44] It is also frequently of value in the postoperative evaluation of patients (Fig. 2-23).

ERP is of particular value when symptoms recur or there is a question of persistent obstruction in the ductal system[32] in patients who have undergone sphincteroplasty or pancreatic drainage procedures.

The relative value of retrograde pancreatography versus computed tomography and sonography in the recognition and diagnosis of pancreatic disease has not been adequately investigated. These studies should be regarded as complementary rather than individually exclusive, since false-positive or false-negative findings may occur in any one of them. At present, when a mass lesion of the pancreas is suspected, we prefer computed tomography or sonography as an initial study with pancreatography as a confirmatory procedure when there is some degree of uncertainty about the diagnosis. When chronic pancreatitis is suspected, pancreatography is favored as the initial procedure.

Computed tomography

JOHN R. HAAGA and RALPH J. ALFIDI

The diagnosis of pancreatic diseases has been aided and simplified by computed tomography (CT). This relatively new diagnostic test is based on the amount of attenuation that a roentgen ray undergoes while coursing through body tissues. The principles and technical aspects have been described in detail. For the first time direct visualization of normal and abnormal pancreases by noninvasive methods is practical and accurate.

NORMAL PANCREAS

An exceptionally clear picture of a normal pancreas and peripancreatic area is seen in Fig. 2-24. The head of the normal pancreas overlies the second lumbar vertebra. The tail is angled cephalad and to the left. Therefore more than one cross-sectional view may be necessary to demonstrate the entire pancreas. The head of the gland is surrounded by the stomach and duodenum. The neck and body overlie the superior mesenteric vessels and can be demonstrated because of the surrounding fat planes. The tip of the tail is located near the splenic hilus. Occasionally the portal vein and pancreaticoduodenal artery can be demonstrated.

Diameters of the pancreas relative to the widths of lumbar vertebrae have been used to determine normal dimensions. These measurements, which serve as a guide, are as follows: the diameter of the head should be less than the width of a vertebral body (usually more than half this width); the body and tail should be less than two thirds the vertebral diameter (usually more than one third the diameter).

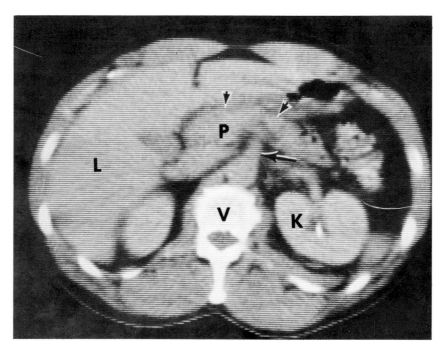

Fig. 2-24. The normal pancreas *(P)* (outlined by arrowheads) lies anterior to the aorta and superior mesenteric artery (large arrow). The liver *(L)* with the proximal portion of the gallbladder is well seen. The falciform ligament dividing the left lobe is clearly visible. The left kidney *(K)* and a lumbar vertebra *(V)* are useful reference points. (From Haaga, J. R., et al.: Radiology **124**:723, 1977.)

PANCREATIC NEOPLASMS

One great advantage of CT has been in the evaluation of jaundiced patients suspected of having a neoplasm, particularly when intravenous cholangiography is certain to be ineffective.

In many instances a mass lesion of the pancreas or periampullary area can be visualized (Figs. 2-25, 2-26, and 2-28). Invasion or encroachment of contiguous structures may also be seen. Besides these direct signs, indirect evidence of obstruction (by tumor, stone, or inflammation) includes dilatation of the intrahepatic and extrahepatic biliary tree (Fig. 2-27). Occasionally indirect evidence is the only suggestion of a small periampullary tumor. Dilatation of the biliary tree is demonstrated because the bile-filled ducts are less dense than the surrounding hepatic parenchyma. At times the dilated ducts extend to the periphery of the liver and can be confused with intrahepatic cysts (Fig. 2-27).

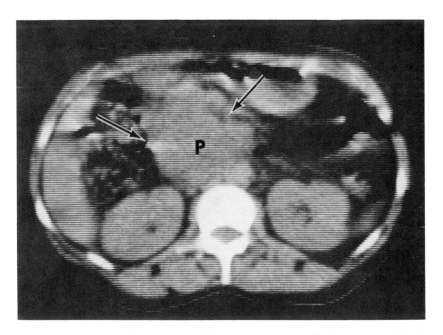

Fig. 2-25. Adenocarcinoma of the head of the pancreas *(P)*. This large tumor is obscuring the fat planes around the aorta and has spread outside the pancreas. Arrows point to boundaries of the tumor. (From Haaga, J. R., et al.: Radiology **124:**723, 1977.)

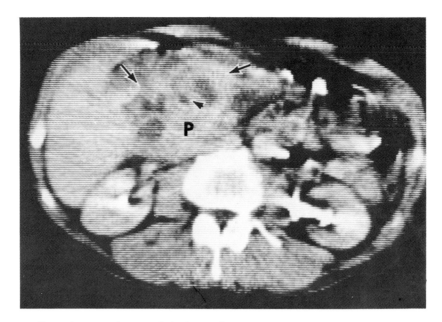

Fig. 2-26. Cystadenocarcinoma of the head of the pancreas *(P)*. This large mass has areas of decreased density throughout the pancreas. These areas are mucin deposits. Arrows point to the mucin. (From Haaga, J. R., et al.: Radiology **124**:723, 1977.)

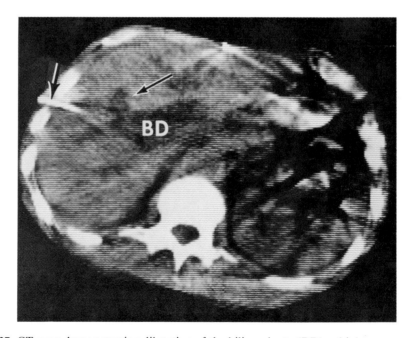

Fig. 2-27. CT scan demonstrating dilatation of the biliary ducts *(BD)*, which appear as areas of decreased density (darker areas) with a branching configuration. Large arrow points to a needle being guided for biliary drainage.

PANCREATITIS

CT in acute pancreatitis of any cause may show diffuse or focal enlargement of the gland. Although edema of the gland has been reported to lower the attenuation numbers (i.e., cause a decrease in density on the CT scan), we have not confirmed this. Since the presence of an enlarged pancreas does not correlate with serum amylase levels, it is difficult to know what percentage of patients with acute pancreatitis will have an enlarged gland. Abscesses or pseudocysts in the lesser sac may also be detected (Figs. 2-30 and 2-31).

In chronic pancreatitis the pancreas may be of normal, small, or increased size. When calcium is deposited in the parenchyma or ducts, it can be visualized by CT scans (Figs. 2-32 and 2-33).

Cystic collections of fluid within or around the pancreas are usually due to pseudocysts. Both the location and the size of these pseudocysts may be visualized.

CT-GUIDED BIOPSIES

CT guidance for percutaneous biopsy has been used in many intra-abdominal diseases (particularly for metastatic lesions). With a symptomatic neoplasm of the body of the pancreas, successful percutaneous fine needle biopsies have been diagnostic and spared the patient an operation.

In selected patients who are terminally ill and become jaundiced, we have employed the CT scanner to decompress the main biliary radicles and liver. This is done by a guided percutaneous technique (Fig. 2-27).

PERSPECTIVE

Where CT fits in the diagnostic evaluation of patients with pancreatic disease remains unclear. Its noninvasive technique and high degree of acceptance have made it a popular test. Prospective studies are necessary; but we suspect that, despite some false-positive and false-negative scans and interpretations, it will be employed universally when mass lesions are suspected. Its use in pancreatitis is probably limited.

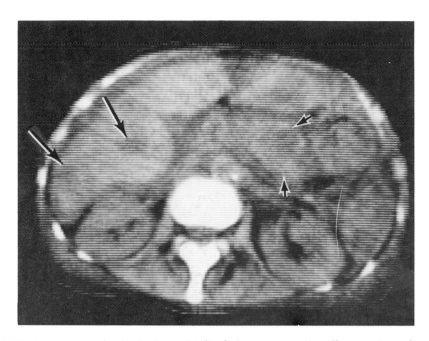

Fig. 2-28. Large mass in the body and tail of the pancreas (small arrows) produced by adenocarcinoma. Note the multiple areas of decreased density throughout the liver (large arrows). These represent metastases. (From Haaga, J. R., et al.: Radiology **124:**723, 1977.)

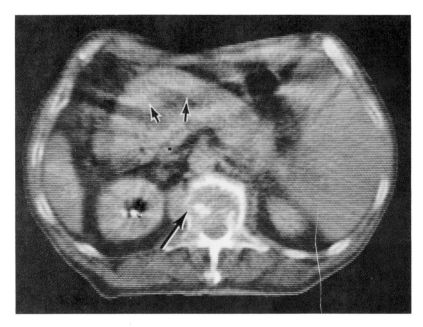

Fig. 2-29. Metastatic adenocarcinoma to the retroperitoneum anteriorly displacing the pancreas. Small arrows are in the pancreas. There is also a metastasis present within the bone (large arrow). (From Haaga, J. R., et al.: Radiology **124:**723, 1977.)

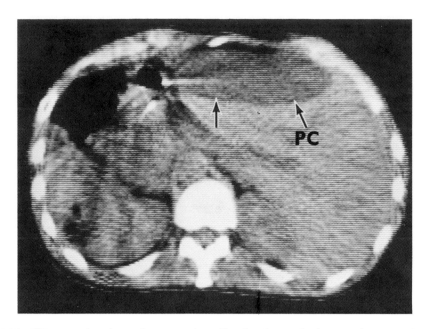

Fig. 2-30. CT scan showing a large cystic collection beneath the anterior capsule of the liver. This later proved to be a pseudocyst *(PC)*. Arrows point to the pseudocyst. (From Haaga, J. R., et al.: Radiology **124**:723, 1977.)

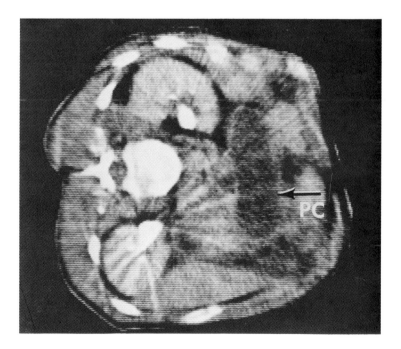

Fig. 2-31. Large mass in the area of the pancreas. CT scan confirms that this is a pseudocyst *(PC)* and not a solid mass. Arrow points to the pseudocyst. (From Haaga, J. R., et al.: Radiology **124**:723, 1977.)

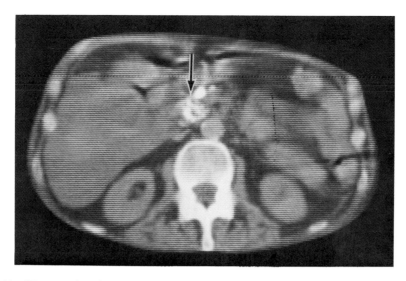

Fig. 2-32. CT scan showing calcific pancreatitis. Multiple calcifications are present within the head of the pancreas (arrow). (From Haaga, J. R., et al.: Radiology, **124:**723, 1977.)

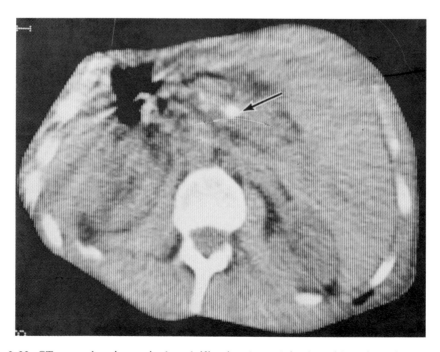

Fig. 2-33. CT scan showing a single calcification (arrow) in the midportion of the head of the pancreas. This was diagnosed as a pancreatic duct calculus and confirmed at surgery. (From Haaga, J. R., et al.: Radiology **124:**723, 1977.)

Angiography

NORBERT E. REICH and THOMAS R. HAVRILLA

The diagnosis of pancreatic disease, in particular the diagnosis of pancreatic carcinoma, has always posed a difficult problem. Despite recent advances in radiology, the pancreas remains a difficult organ to examine. Current roentgenographic methods to evaluate the pancreas include conventional roentgenography, ultrasonography, radionuclide imaging, pancreatography, computed tomography, and angiography. Of these modalities, selective and superselective pancreatic angiography offers the greatest specificity for examination of the pancreas.

METHOD OF EXAMINATION

A preshaped no. 5 or 7 French catheter is percutaneously introduced into the femoral artery using the technique described by Seldinger.[72] If iliofemoral occlusive disease is present, the catheter may be introduced into a branchial or axillary artery. The preshaped catheter is then selectively advanced into the celiac and superior mesenteric arteries separately. After injection of the contrast agent, serial films are obtained in the arterial, capillary, and venous phases of the contrast circulation. Direct 2× serial magnification and superselective injection into the gastroduodenal, pancreatic branches of the splenic, or superior mesenteric artery may then be performed if warranted on the basis of the findings of celiac and superior mesenteric arteriograms or by the clinical setting. Moreover, pharmacoangiography plays an important role in the evaluation of pancreatic disease. Vasoconstrictive agents such as epinephrine, norepinephrine, vasopressin, and angiotensin or vasodilators such as bradykinin and tolazoline, or a combination of vasoconstrictors and vasodilators, may be used to improve visualization of both normal and abnormal pancreatic vascular anatomy.[58,60,76] Stimulation by secretin, histamine, or trypsin may improve visualization of the parenchymal phase of the pancreatic arteriogram.[71]

More recently emphasis has been placed on the venous phase of the pancreatic arteriogram as an early and more sensitive indicator of pancreatic disease.[52] In the event that the venous anatomy is not well visualized despite the use of pharmacologic agents, splenoportography or selective catheterization of pancreatic veins by transhepatic portal catheterization via jugular and hepatic veins or umbilical veins may be accomplished.[56,69]

NORMAL VASCULAR ANATOMY

The blood supply to the pancreas is derived from the celiac and the superior mesenteric arteries. The celiac trunk divides into the common hepatic, splenic, and left gastric arteries (Fig. 2-34). The major portion of

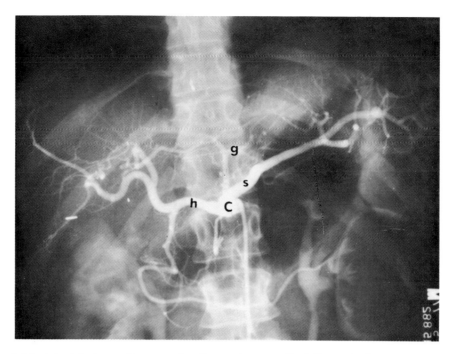

Fig. 2-34. Arterial phase of a normal celiac angiogram. *C*, Celiac axis; *h*, common hepatic artery; *s*, splenic artery; *g*, left gastric artery.

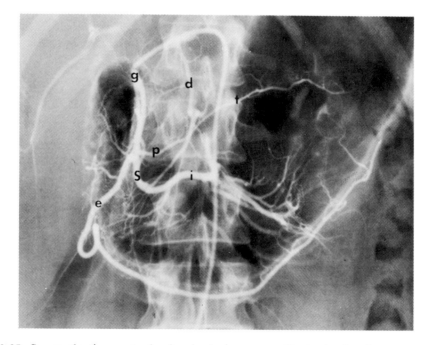

Fig. 2-35. Superselective gastroduodenal arteriogram. *g*, Gastroduodenal artery; *e*, right gastroepiploic artery; *S*, superior anterior pancreaticoduodenal artery; *i*, inferior anterior pancreaticoduodenal artery; *p*, posterior superior pancreaticoduodenal artery; *d*, dorsal pancratic artery; *t*, transverse pancreatic artery.

the blood supply to the pancreas comes from the hepatic artery, splenic artery, and superior mesenteric artery.

The gastroduodenal artery, the first major branch of the hepatic artery, courses behind the first portion of the duodenum (Fig. 2-35). The *posterior superior pancreaticoduodenal artery* is its first branch. This artery passes along the dorsal surface of the head of the pancreas, supplying the pancreatic head, and then anastomoses with the posterior inferior pancreaticoduodenal artery (which arises from the superior mesenteric artery) to form the posterior arcade. The second branch of the gastroduodenal artery, the *anterior superior pancreaticoduodenal artery,* passes over the anterior surface of the head of the pancreas and also supplies the pancreatic head. The anterior inferior pancreaticoduodenal artery, a branch of the superior mesenteric artery, joins with the anterior superior pancreaticoduodenal artery to form the anterior arcade.

The splenic artery, coursing to the left from the celiac artery, gives off many branches to the body and the tail of the pancreas. A major branch, the *dorsal pancreatic artery,* arises from the proximal portion of the splenic artery. It passes caudally into the body of the pancreas. Here it branches into the *transverse pancreatic artery,* which supplies both the head and the tail of the pancreas. The tail of the pancreas is also supplied by the *pancreatica magna artery,* arising from the distal portion of the

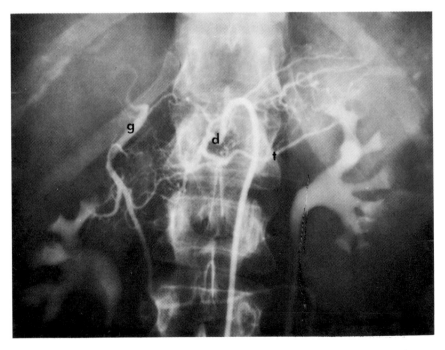

Fig. 2-36. Superselective dorsal pancreatic arteriogram. *d,* Dorsal pancreatic artery; *t,* transverse pancreatic artery; *g,* gastroduodenal artery.

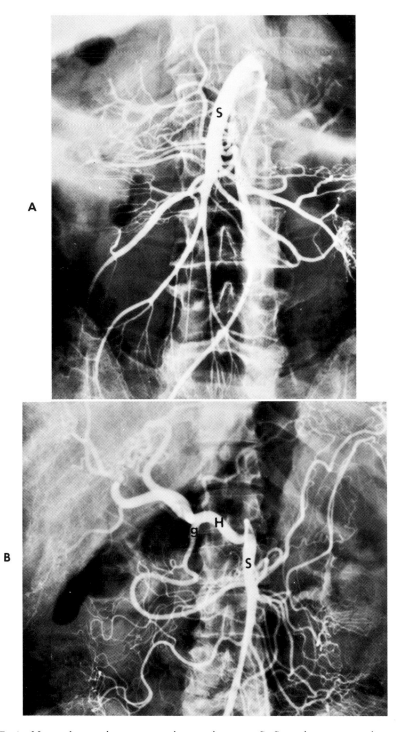

Fig. 2-37. A, Normal superior mesenteric arteriogram. *S,* Superior mesenteric artery. **B,** Normal variant of a superior mesenteric arteriogram. The entire blood supply to the liver is derived from the superior mesenteric artery *(S). H,* Common hepatic artery; *g,* gastroduodenal artery.

splenic artery. Many small pancreatic vessels arise from the left gastroepiploic artery and from the terminal branches of the splenic artery to supply the tail of the pancreas.

The arterial supply to the pancreas is variable, and often superselective angiography is necessary to evaluate the intrapancreatic arteries (Figs. 2-35 and 2-36). Of particular note, the *hepatic artery* may arise entirely from the superior mesenteric artery (14% of the population) (Fig. 2-37, *B*). Then the whole circulation to the duodenum and liver originates from the *superior mesenteric artery.* Under these circumstances pancreaticoduodenectomy may be difficult without sacrificing the hepatic vessels and perhaps necrosing the liver. An *accessory right hepatic artery* may arise from the superior mesenteric artery (approximately 8% of the population) (Fig. 2-38). Furthermore, the numerous variations, locations, and tortuosity of the *splenic artery* may lead to its being found either inferior or superior to the midportion of the pancreas. For these reasons patients in whom extensive resective surgery of the pancreas is contemplated should

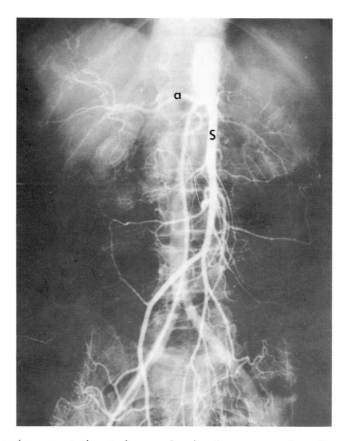

Fig. 2-38. Superior mesenteric arteriogram showing the accessory hepatic artery *(a)* originating from the superior mesenteric artery *(S)* and supplying part of the liver.

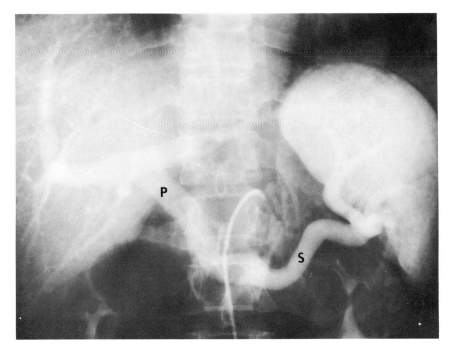

Fig. 2-39. Venous phase of a celiac arteriogram. *P*, Portal vein; *S*, splenic vein.

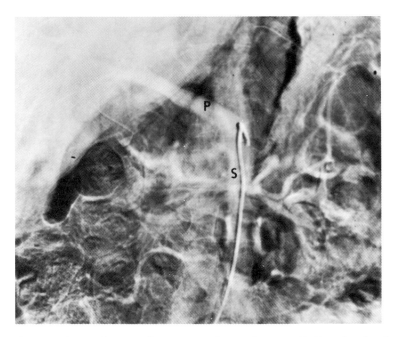

Fig. 2-40. Venous phase of a superior mesenteric arteriogram. *S*, superior mesenteric vein.

undergo selective angiography of the celiac and superior mesenteric vessels.

The venous system is also variable, but knowledge of its anatomy and drainage patterns is important for a thorough angiographic investigation. The veins of the gastrointestinal tract drain into the portal system. The superior mesenteric vein and the splenic vein join to form the portal vein. The portal vein then enters the liver hilum and divides into right and left branches which empty toward the periphery of the liver (Figs. 2-39 and 2-40).

INDICATIONS FOR PANCREATIC ANGIOGRAPHY

Pancreatic angiography not only helps to establish the diagnosis but is a prerequisite in some patients with known pancreatic disease in whom surgical intervention is contemplated. The arteriogram aids differentiating between inflammatory disease and carcinoma of the pancreas. Preoperatively the arteriogram defines the vascular anatomy for the surgeon. Location of the tumor, extent of the disease, and resectability can also be predicted on the basis of the arteriographic findings. These findings correlate with operability and survival.[74,75]

COMPLICATIONS OF ARTERIOGRAPHY

When evaluating diagnostic usefulness, as with any procedure, the examiner must consider potential risks. With experience, complications are few. Minor complications occur in less than 3%, and major complications in less than 0.5%, of patients.[65] Included are complications occurring at the site of catheter introduction and those secondary to catheter manipulation. In the former group are bleeding, femoral artery thrombosis, and less commonly arteriovenous fistulae, pseudoaneurysms, embolization of blood clot or atherosclerotic plaque to the leg, thrombophlebitis, local dissection of the femoral artery, and the development of infection. Complications resulting from catheter manipulation include dissection of the aorta or its branches, vascular perforation, wedging of the catheter (which may produce chemotoxic or ischemic damage), intravascular breakage of the catheter and guide wires, and embolization of atherosclerotic debris.[62]

DIAGNOSTIC CRITERIA
Pancreatitis

Although pancreatic angiography is rarely used as a primary diagnostic procedure with pancreatitis, arteriographic changes must be understood to differentiate it from carcinoma of the pancreas. There is confusion in the literature concerning the arteriographic findings of pancreatitis. Reported

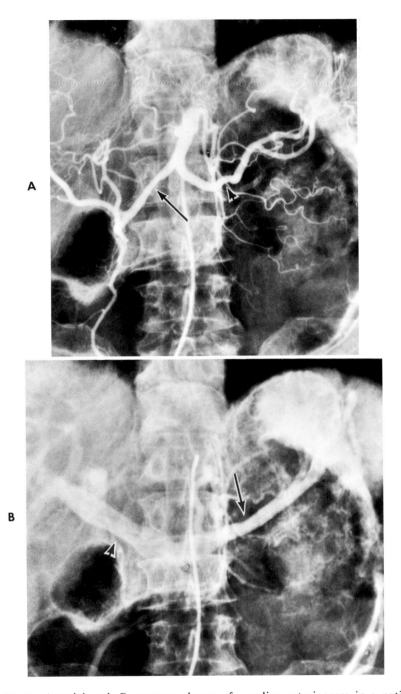

Fig. 2-41. A, Arterial and, **B,** venous phases of a celiac arteriogram in a patient with pancreatitis. Smooth encasement of the common hepatic artery (**A,** arrow) and splenic artery (**A,** arrowhead) and of the portal vein (**B,** arrowhead) and splenic vein (**B,** arrow) is evident.

angiographic findings include normal vascular anatomy, enlargement of the pancreas, hypovascularity and hypervascularity, and smooth and irregular encasement of intrapancreatic and surrounding arteries and veins (Fig. 2-41).[63,64,68,69]

The arteriographic findings, no doubt, are related to the severity and duration of the pancreatitis. Acute pancreatitis may show no specific findings. If the pancreas is edematous, the vessels may be attenuated and the pancreas appear hypervascular. Recurrent disease results in arterial irregularities of the intrapancreatic branches. The parenchyma may become prominently hypervascular. With increasing fibrosis, as in chronic pancreatitis, the major intrapancreatic arteries assume a beaded appearance (Fig. 2-42), and aneurysm formation (though rare) may be a specific sign of pancreatitis. The aneurysms are believed to result from the release of pancreatic enzymes, causing weakening of the vessel walls. In this stage of the disease, the major vessels surrounding the pancreas also may become narrowed. Despite the high degree of accuracy reported by Goldstein and co-workers[55] in the differential diagnosis of pancreatitis from carcinoma of the pancreas, it is generally agreed that such differential diagnosis may be quite difficult.

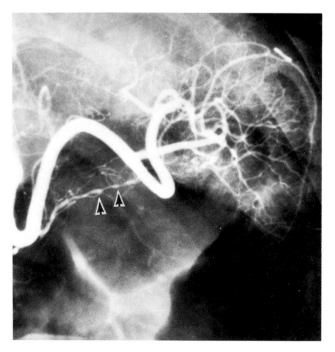

Fig. 2-42. Beaded appearance of the transverse pancreatic artery (arrowheads) in a patient with chronic pancreatitis. The venous phase of the arteriogram showed no abnormality.

Pseudocysts

Pancreatic pseudocysts usually result from pancreatitis or trauma to the pancreas. Arteriographically, small pseudocysts cause stretching of intrapancreatic vessels. Larger cysts may also cause displacement of the splenic, hepatic, or gastroduodenal and mesenteric arteries (Fig. 2-43). During the capillary phase a filling defect is observed. Large pseudocysts may result in occlusion of the splenic vein. On occasion, it is difficult to differentiate a pseudocyst from an atypical avascular cystadenoma.

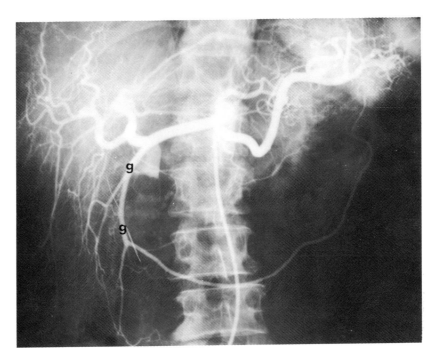

Fig. 2-43. The gastroduodenal artery *(g)* is stretched around a large pseudocyst located in the head of the pancreas. Note the presence of pancreatic calcifications.

Carcinoma of the pancreas

Arteriography plays a primary role in the diagnosis of carcinoma of the pancreas. It also enables the surgeon to evaluate the extent, resectability, and curability of the disease. According to different series the prospective accuracy of angiographic diagnosis of carcinoma of the pancreas varies from 50% to 94%.* A high degree of accuracy is obtained by utilizing superselective injections as well as pharmacoangiography.

As with other infiltrating malignancies of the gastrointestinal tract, adenocarcinoma of the pancreas is poorly vascularized. The primary angiographic abnormality is encasement of intrapancreatic or adjacent large arteries (Fig. 2-44). The type of encasement ranges from the virtually pathognomic serrated or serpiginous form (Fig. 2-45) to the less specific smooth narrowing which might be difficult to differentiate from atherosclerosis (Figs. 2-46 and 2-47). Smaller intrapancreatic vessels may show abrupt angulation.

Tumor vascularity can be seen in 60% of carcinomas of the pancreas, when superselective techniques are utilized.[67] Buranasiri and Baum[52] have emphasized the importance of the venous phase. Carcinomas in the head of the pancreas may distort or occlude the superior mesenteric or portal

*References 51, 53, 55, 61, 66.

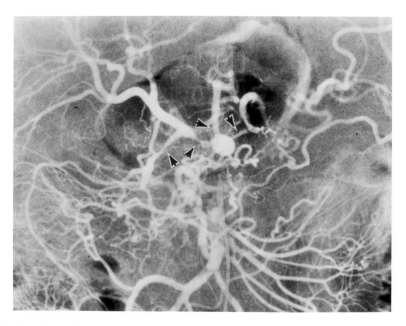

Fig. 2-44. Carcinoma in the head and body of the pancreas causing encasement of the major arteries surrounding the pancreas (arrowheads). The patient also had atherosclerosis and an aneurysm of the celiac artery.

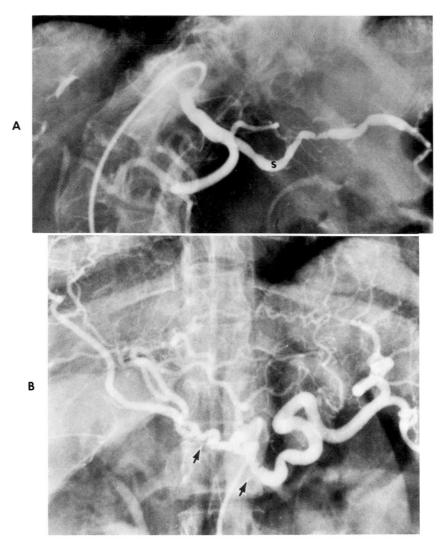

Fig. 2-45. A, Serrated encasement of the splenic artery *(s)* in a patient with carcinoma of the pancreas. **B,** Serrated and serpiginous encasement (arrows) of the splenic and common hepatic arteries characteristic of carcinoma of the pancreas.

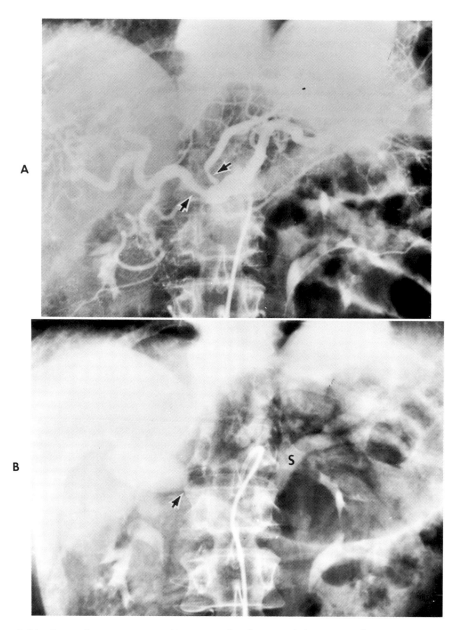

Fig. 2-46. Smooth encasement (**A**, arrows) of several large arteries surrounding the pancreas. This may be difficult to differentiate from atherosclerosis. However, the venous phase of the arteriogram shows abrupt narrowing and distal dilatation of the portal vein (**B**, arrow). The latter finding, in combination with the encasement, helped establish the correct diagnosis of carcinoma of the pancreas. Venous involvement is not observed in atherosclerosis. *S*, Splenic vein.

vein (Fig. 2-46, *B*); those located in the tail of the pancreas may cause narrowing or occlusion of the splenic vein (Fig. 2-48). Arterial displacement, early venous drainage, and vascular staining are unusual findings with carcinoma of the pancreas. More characteristically, sparse filling during the arterial and capillary phase may be observed.[53]

In outlining the vascular anatomy for the surgeon, the pancreatic arteriogram not only helps to establish the diagnosis but also is useful for determining the resectability of the tumor. Encasement of the celiac, superior mesenteric, hepatic, gastric, or intestinal arteries, invasion or occlusion of portal or superior mesenteric veins, and hepatic metastases are signs of nonresectability. Invasion of only one or two intrapancreatic arteries may be correlated with resectability and survival, particularly when the tumors are located in the head of the pancreas.[74,75]

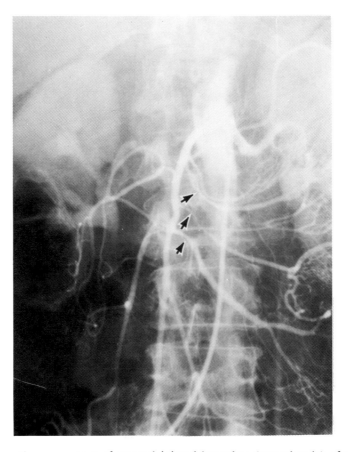

Fig. 2-47. Smooth encasement of several jejunal branches (arrowheads) of the superior mesenteric artery in a patient with atherosclerosis. The venous phase of the arteriogram was normal.

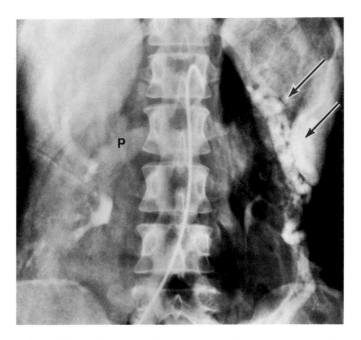

Fig. 2-48. Occlusion of the splenic vein in a patient with pancreatic carcinoma. Note the absence of a normal splenic vein and the abundant collateral veins (arrows). *P,* Portal vein.

Endocrine tumors of the pancreas

Secreting endocrine tumors can usually be detected clinically, but their exact location within the pancreas is of great importance. Surgical removal results in cure, but their small size makes identification at surgery difficult. Surgical success in removing these tumors blindly is only 50%.[77] Preoperative localization by angiography therefore plays an important role in the management of these tumors.

Examinations of high technical quality result in accuracy of greater than 90%.[54] Furthermore, selective catheterization of the pancreatic veins for hormone assay may prove to be a valuable adjunct in the localization of functioning endocrine tumors of the pancreas.[59] Angiographic findings include a hypervascular arterial phase, draining veins, and tumor staining (Fig. 2-49). The lesions are usually well circumscribed. In the absence of liver metastases, angiography cannot differentiate between benign and malignant tumors.

Nonfunctioning islet cell tumors are also hypervascular and exhibit a dense capillary stain. Unlike the functioning variety, however, neovascularity is not uncommon. At time of diagnosis, these tumors tend to be larger than their functioning counterpart probably because of the lack of clinical symptoms (Fig. 2-50).[50]

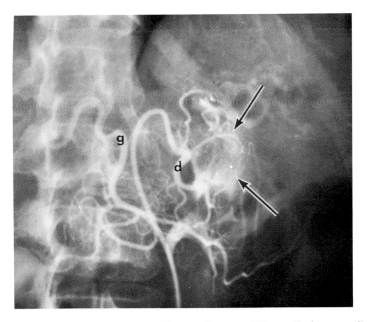

Fig. 2-49. Superselective dorsal pancreatic arteriogram. The well-circumscribed tumor-stained vascular mass (arrows) represents a functioning islet cell adenoma. *g*, Gastroduodenal artery; *d*, dorsal pancreatic artery.

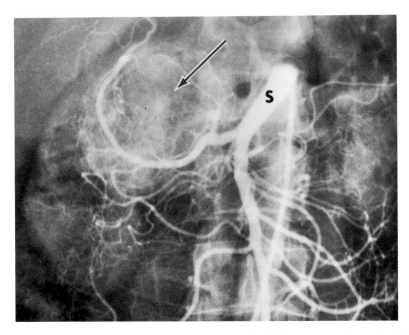

Fig. 2-50. Large vascular islet cell adenoma in the head of the pancreas (arrow). *S*, Superior mesenteric artery.

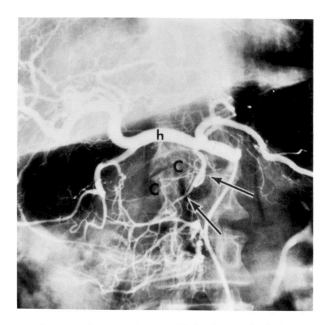

Fig. 2-51. Hypovascular cystadenocarcinoma *(C)* in the head of the pancreas attenuating and displaying the intrapancreatic arteries (arrows) as well as the common hepatic artery *(h).*

Cystadenoma and cystadenocarcinoma

These lesions are relatively rare primary neoplasms of the pancreas. The classic angiographic findings include a vascular mass, large feeding arteries, displacement of major vessels, and prominent tumor blush. At the time of angiography, it is not possible to differentiate benign and malignant cystadenomas. Malignancy must be suspected when the lesion is large. Occasionally pancreatic cystadenocarcinomas are hypovascular and are then indistinguishable from pancreatic pseudocysts (Fig. 2-51).

Trauma

Few descriptions of the angiographic appearance of pancreatic trauma are available.[57,73] Angiographic features include occlusion of pancreatic arteries and impairment of the arterial circulation. The presence of a hematoma may lead to displacement of adjacent arteries or veins.

CONCLUSION

Pancreatic angiography can play a major role in the diagnosis of pancreatic disease and also in the evaluation of the extent of the disease, in the preoperative localization, in the prediction of resectability and curability, and in the demonstration of the vascular anatomy. Meticulous technique, superselective catheterization, and the use of pharmacoangiography produce a high degree of accuracy in the hands of experienced angiographers.

Ultrasonography

LEOPOLD GONZALEZ and SEBASTIAN A. COOK

Ultrasonography is a relatively new, noninvasive, method of studying the pancreas. Ultrasound relies on differences in physical characteristics of the various organs through which sound travels to produce images of the objects studied. It provides the examiner an opportunity to appreciate any variations in the physical relationships of the normal organs as well as detect intrinsic change within an organ itself. No ionizing radiation is involved. With the introduction and refinement of the gray scale scanners, there has been increasing use of ultrasound in evaluating pancreatic disorders.

No universally employed technique for scanning the pancreas exists. Many investigators, however, utilize the supine position to study the head and body of the pancreas with longitudinal and oblique scans; they have also found that in the prone position scanning through the upper pole of the left kidney helps evaluate the tail of the pancreas. Most investigators initially thought the pancreas itself could not be visualized. More recently they have become convinced that pancreatic tissue can be identified, but they still rely on surrounding vascular and biliary structures to help identify the pancreatic region.[83]

Filly and Freimanis[81] diagrammatically and with actual case material vividly depicted the major abdominal vessels used to localize the pancreas. The splenic artery courses along the superior border of the pancreas whereas the splenic vein is the posterior boundary. The superior mesenteric artery, frequently seen on a transverse section in the center of a tent-shaped echo-rich area, also serves as a guidepost in identifying the region of the pancreas. Typically the pancreas has internal echoes which are brighter than those of the liver though not as dense as those in connective tissue (Fig. 2-52).

The pancreas becomes edematous in acute pancreatitis and echographically more sonolucent, showing fewer echoes than the liver. Splenic and portal veins are usually not identified as separate structures. Because no strict criteria exist for diagnosing acute pancreatitis, the accuracy in diagnosing this disorder echographically is difficult to know. Weill and co-workers[86] reported their accuracy as 91%, and Hancke[83] as 82%, in this disorder though Doust and Pearce,[79] using more refined objective criteria, reported a diagnostic accuracy rate of approximately 80%.

Pancreatic abscesses and pseudocysts, complications of pancreatitis, are more easily diagnosed than acute pancreatitis. Lower limits of resolution are in the range of 2 to 3 cm diameter. If there is debris within the cyst, however, it can be difficult to decide whether one is dealing with a solid mass or a partially fluid-filled structure. Reported series range from 87% to 100% accuracy in diagnosing pancreatic pseudocysts (Fig. 2-53).[78,82,84]

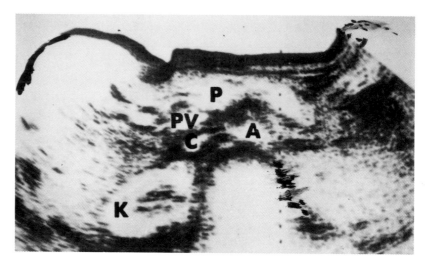

Fig. 2-52. Transverse section of the upper abdomen demonstrating a normal-appearing pancreas *(P)*. Other abdominal structures are the portal vein *(PV)*, vena cava *(C)*, abdominal aorta *(A)*, and right kidney *(K)*.

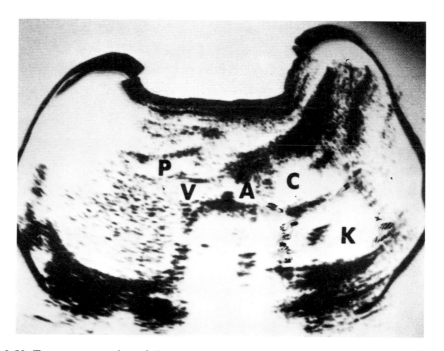

Fig. 2-53. Transverse section of the upper abdomen demonstrating a pseudocyst *(C)* of the pancreas anterior to the left kidney *(K)*. Other structures are the portal vein *(P)*, vena cava *(V)*, and abdominal aorta *(A)*.

Chronic pancreatitis may be recognized by the presence of cystic areas and calcifications in the region of the pancreas. These are due to dilated ducts or small cysts. Areas of fibrosis may be present, showing as increased echoes, which cannot be differentiated from infiltrating carcinoma.

Carcinoma of the pancreas is usually seen as a mass lesion with a solid appearance. Not uncommonly it is associated with secondary pancreatitis, in which case differentiating is obviously impossible (Fig. 2-54).

Differences in diagnostic criteria, patient selection, and equipment utilized contribute to making it unrealistic to draw any conclusions about the effectiveness of ultrasonography in pancreatic tumor diagnosis. Nevertheless, several authors have reported their experiences.[78,80]

Clinical factors (including the patient's condition, obesity, ascites, and the presence of abdominal gas) limit the usefulness of ultrasound in diagnosing all pancreatic disorders.

By way of summary, ultrasound provides a noninvasive method of studying the pancreas. With improved technology, particularly in utilization of the gray scale, there has been a significant improvement in the clinical applicability and accuracy of ultrasound.[85] There is reason to believe that further developments will continue to increase the clinical value of this modality in diagnosing pancreatic disease.

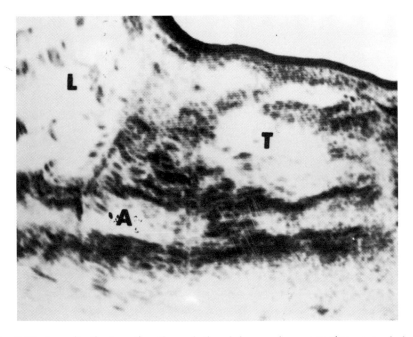

Fig. 2-54. Longitudinal section through the abdomen demonstrating an oval-shaped tumor mass in the pancreas *(T)*. Note the presence of internal echoes, which helps to identify this as a solid mass. Liver *(L)* and aorta *(A)* are also identified.

REFERENCES
Conventional roentgenographic diagnosis

 1. Baylin, G. J., and Weeks, K. D.: Some roentgen aspects of pancreatic necrosis, Radiology **42**:466, 1944.
 2. Berenson, J. E., Spitz, H. B., and Felson, B.: The abdominal fat necrosis sign, Radiology **100**:567, 1971.
 3. Brascho, D. J., and Reynolds, R. N.: The radiographic "colon cut-off sign" in acute pancreatitis, Radiology **79**:763, 1962.
 4. Cantwell, D. E., and Pollock, A. V.: Radiology of acute pancreatitis, J. Fac. Radiol. **10**:95, 1959.
 5. Eaton, S. B., Jr., and Ferrucci, J. T., Jr.: Radiology of the pancreas and duodenum, Philadelphia, 1973, W. B. Saunders Co.
 6. Felson, B.: Gas abscess of the pancreas, J.A.M.A. **163**:637, 1957.
 7. Felson, B.: Letter from the editor, Semin. Roentgenol. **3**:215, 1968.
 8. Fishbein, R., Murphy, G. P., and Wilder, R. J.: The pleuropulmonary manifestations of pancreatitis, Dis. Chest **41**:392, 1962.
 9. Geokas, M.D., VanLanckner, J.L., Kadell, B. M., and Machleder, H. I.: Acute pancreatitis—UCLA conference, Ann. Intern. Med. **76**:105, 1972.
10. Goldstein, H. M., and Zboralske, F. F.: Tubeless hypotonic duodenography, J.A.M.A. **210**:2086, 1969.
11. Gorder, J. L., and Stargardter, F. L.: Pancreatic pseudotumors simulating intrarenal masses, Am. J. Roentgenol. Radium Ther. Nucl. Med. **107**:65, 1969.
12. Jacquemet, P., Liotta, D., and Mallet, G. P.: The early radiologic diagnosis of diseases of the pancreas and ampulla of Vater, Springfield, Ill., 1965, Charles C Thomas, Publisher.
13. Kattwinkel, J., Ladey, A., deSant'Agnese, P. A., Edwards, W. A., and Juffy, M. P.: Hereditary pancreatitis: three new kindreds and a critical review of the literature, Pediatrics **51**:55, 1973.
14. Lipp, W. E., and Aaron, A. H.: Acute pancreatitis: further observations of value in its recognition, N.Y. State J. Med. **50**:2043, 1950.
15. Mani, J. R., Zboralski, F. F., and Margulis, A. R.: Carcinoma of the body and tail of the pancreas, Am. J. Roentgenol. Radium Ther. Nucl. Med. **96**:429, 1966.
16. Martel, W., Scholtens, P. A., and Lim, L. W.: Tubeless hypotonic duodenography: technique, value and limitations, Am. J. Roentgenol. Radium Ther. Nucl. Med. **107**:119, 1969.
17. McClintock, J. T., McFee, J. L., and Quimby, R. L.: Pancreatic pseudocyst presenting as a mediastinal tumor, J.A.M.A. **192**:573, 1965.
18. Minagi, H., and Hargolin, F. R.: Pancreatic calcifications, Am. J. Gastroenterol. **57**:139, 1972.
19. Nelson, S. W., and Christoforidis, A. J.: Roentgenologic features of the Zollinger-Ellison syndrome: ulcerogenic tumor of the pancreas, Semin. Roentgenol. **3**:254, 1968.
20. Price, C. W. R.: The colon cut-off sign in acute pancreatitis, Med. J. Aust. **1**:313, 1956.
21. Roseman, D. M., Konlessar, O. D., and Sleisenger, M. H.: Pulmonary manifestations of pancreatitis, N. Engl. J. Med. **263**:294, 1960.
22. Sarles, H.: Progress in hepatology: chronic calcifying pancreatitis—chronic alcoholic pancreatitis, Gastroenterology **66**:604, 1974.
23. Schindler, S. C., Schaefer, J. W., Hull, D., and Griffen, W. O.: Chronic pancreatic ascites, Gastroenterology **59**:453, 1970.
24. Seaman, W. B., Sorabella, P. A., and Campbell, W. L.: Roentgen detection of enlarge-

ment of the body and tail of the pancreas using the supine translateral projection, Radiology **111:**529, 1974.

25. Sibert, J. R.: A British family with hereditary pancreatitis, Gut **16:**81, 1975.
26. Sorabella, P. A., Campbell, W. L., and Seaman, W. B.: The axial pancreatic view: a new approach for recognizing enlargement of the body and tail of the pancreas, Radiology **111:**535, 1974.
27. Stein, G. N., Kalser, M. H., Sapian, N. N., and Finkelstein, A.: An evaluation of the roentgen changes in acute pancreatitis: correlation with clinical findings, Gastroenterology **36:**354, 1959.
28. Weens, H. S., and Walker, L. A.: The radiologic diagnosis of acute cholecystitis and pancreatitis, Radiol. Clin. North Am. **2:**89, 1964.
29. Wilson, T. S., and Costopoulos, L. B.: The diagnosis and treatment of pancreatic pseudocysts, Can. Med. Assoc. J. **97:**1117, 1967.

Endoscopic retrograde cholangiopancreatography

30. Bilbao, M. K., Dotter, C. T., Lee, T. G., and Katon, R. M.: Complications of endoscopic retrograde cholangiopancreatography (ERCP). A study of 10,000 cases, Gastroenterology **70:**314, 1976.
31. Braasch, J. W., and Gregg, J. A.: Surgical uses of peroral retrograde pancreatography and cholangiography, Am. J. Surg. **125:**432, 1973.
32. Cooperman, A. M., Sivak, M. V., Sullivan, B. H., Jr., and Hermann, R. E.: Endoscopic pancreatography. Its value in preoperative and postoperative assessment of pancreatic disease, Am. J. Surg. **129:**38, 1975.
33. Cotton, P. B., and Beales, J. S.: Endoscopic pancreatography in management of relapsing acute pancreatitis, Br. Med. J. **1:**608, 1974.
34. Doubilet, H., Poppel, M. H., and Mulholland, J. H.: Pancreatography. Technics, principles, and observations, Radiology **64:**325, 1955.
35. Howard, J. M., and Nedwich, A.: Correlation of the histologic observations and operative findings in patients with chronic pancreatitis, Surg. Gynecol. Obstet. **132:**387, 1971.
36. Kawanishi, H., Sell, J. E., and Pollard, H. M.: Combined endoscopic pancreatic fluid collection and retrograde pancreatography in the diagnosis of pancreatic cancer and chronic pancreatitis, Gastrointest. Endosc. **22:**82, 1975.
37. Kozower, M., Norton, R. A., Paul, R. E., Jr., Fawaz, K. A., Miller, H. H., Robbins, A. H., Schimmel, E. M., Sugarman, H. J., and Tomas, J. G.: Preoperative endoscopic cannulation of pancreatic and biliary ducts, Ann. Surg. **178:**197, 1973.
38. McCune, W. S., Shorb, P. E., and Moscovitz, H.: Endoscopic cannulation of the ampulla of Vater. A preliminary report, Ann. Surg. **167:**752, 1968.
39. Nakano, S., Horiguchi, Y., Takeda, T., Suzuki, T., and Nakajima, S.: Comparative diagnostic value of endoscopic pancreatography and pancreatic function tests, Scand. J. Gastroenterol. **9:**383, 1974.
40. Oi, I.: Fiberduodenoscopy and endoscopic pancreatocholangiography, Gastrointest. Endosc. **17:**59, 1970.
41. Rabinov, K. R., and Simon, M.: Peroral cannulation of the ampulla of Vater for direct cholangiography and pancreatography, Radiology **85:**693, 1965.
42. Satake, K., Umeyama, K., Kobayashi, K., Mitani, E., Tatsumi, S., Yamamoto, S., and Howard, J. M.: An evaluation of endoscopic pancreatocholangiography in surgical patients, Surg. Gynecol. Obstet. **140:**349, 1975.
43. Sivak, M. V., Jr., and Sullivan, B. H., Jr.: Endoscopic retrograde pancreatography. Analysis of the normal pancreatogram, Am. J. Dig. Dis. **21:**263, 1976.

44. Sugawa, C., Raouf, R., Bradley, V., Westreich, M., Lucas, C. E., and Walt, A. J.: Peroral endoscopic cholangiography and pancreatography. The surgeon's helper, Arch. Surg. **109:**231, 1974.

Computed tomography

45. Alfidi, R. J., Haaga, J. R., Havrilla, T. R., Pepe, R. G., and Cook, S.: Computed tomography of the liver, Am. J. Roentgenol. Radium Ther. Nucl. Med. **127:**69, 1976.
46. Haaga, J. R., and Alfidi, R. J.: Precise biopsy localization by computed tomography, Radiology **118:**603, 1976.
47. Haaga, J. R., Alfidi, R. J., Havrilla, T. R., Tubbs, R., Gonzalez, L., and Meaney, T. F.: Definitive role of CT scanning of the pancreas; the second year's experience, Radiology **124:**723, 1977.
48. Haaga, J. R., Alfidi, R. J., Zelch, M. G., Meaney, T. F., Boller, M., Gonzalez, L., and Jelden, G.: Computed tomography of the pancreas, Radiology **120:**589, 1976.
49. Reich, N. E., Haaga, J. R., and Havrilla, T. R.: Percutaneous drainage of a dilated biliary system. (Submitted for publication.)

Angiography

50. Baghery, S., Alfidi, R. J., and Zelch, M. Z.: Angiography of non-functioning islet cell tumor of the pancreas, Radiology **119:**57, 1976.
51. Bookstein, J. J., Reuter, S. R., and Martel, W.: Angiographic evaluation of pancreatic carcinoma, Radiology **93:**757, 1969.
52. Buranasiri, S., and Baum, S.: The significance of the venous phase of celiac and superior mesenteric arteriography in evaluating pancreatic carcinoma, Radiology **102:**11, 1972.
53. Eisenberg, H.: Angiography of the pancreas. In Hilal, S. K., editor: Small vessel angiography, St. Louis, 1973, The C. V. Mosby Co.
54. Fulton, R. E., Sheedy, P. F., McIlrath, D. C., and Ferris, D. O.: Preoperative angiographic localization of insulin-producing tumors of the pancreas, Am. J. Roentgenol. Radium Ther. Nucl. Med. **123:**367, 1975.
55. Goldstein, H. M., Neiman, H. L., and Bookstein, J. J.: Angiographic evaluation of pancreatic disease, Radiology **112:**275, 1974.
56. Göthlin, J., Lunderguist, A., and Tylén, U.: Selective phlebography of the pancreas, Acta Radiol. [Diagn.] **15:**474, 1974.
57. Haertel, M., and Fuchs, W. A., Angiography in pancreatic trauma, Br. J. Radiol. **47:**641, 1974.
58. Hawkins, I. F., Jr., Kaude, J. V., and MacGregor, A.: Priscoline and epinephrine in selective pancreatic angiography, Radiology **116:**311, 1975.
59. Ingemansson, S., Lunderguist, A., and Holst, J.: Selective catheterization of the pancreatic vein for radioimmunoassay in glucagon secreting carcinoma of the pancreas, Radiology **119:**555, 1976.
60. Kaplan, J. H., and Bookstein, J. J.: Abnormal visceral pharmacoangiography with angiotensin, Radiology **103:**79, 1972.
61. Lunderguist, A.: Angiography in carcinoma of the pancreas, Acta Radiol. [Diagn.], supp. 235, 1965.
62. Meaney T. F.: Complications of percutaneous femoral angiography, Geriatrics **29:**61, 1974.
63. Moskowitz, H., Chait, A., and Mellins, H. Z.: Tumor encasement of the celiac axis due to chronic pancreatitis, Am. J. Roentgenol. Radium Ther. Nucl. Med. **104:**641, 1968.
64. Nebesar R. A., and Pollard, J. J.: A critical evaluation of selective celiac and superior

mesenteric angiography in the diagnosis of pancreatic diseases, particularly malignant tumor: facts and "artefacts," Radiology **89**:1017, 1967.

65. Ranninger, K., and Beachley, M.C.: Pancreatic angiography, Curr. Probl. Radiol. **4**:2, 1974.
66. Ranninger, K., and Saldino, R. M.: Arteriographic diagnosis of pancreatic lesions, Radiology **86**:470, 1966.
67. Reuter, S. R., and Redman, H. C.: Gastrointestinal angiography, Philadelphia, 1972, W. B. Saunders Co.
68. Reuter, S. R., Redman, H. C., and Joseph, R. R.: Angiographic findings in pancreatitis, Am. J. Roentgenol. Radium Ther. Nucl. Med. **107**:56, 1969.
69. Rosch J., Bert, J.: Arteriography of the pancreas, Am. J. Roentgenol. Radium Ther. Nucl. Med. **94**:182, 1965.
70. Rosch, J., and Dotter, C. T.: Retrograde pancreatic venography, Radiology **114**:275, 1975.
71. Schmarsow, R.: Angiography of the pancreas following the administration of secretin, trypsin, and histamine, Acta Radiol. [Diagn.] **12**:175, 1972.
72. Seldinger, S. I.: Catheter replacement of needle in percutaneous arteriography: new technique, Acta Radiol. **39**:368, 1953.
73. Siroudi, M., and Bookstein, J. J.: Angiography in acute pancreatic transection, Radiology **115**:309, 1975.
74. Suzuki, T., Kawabe, K., Imamura, M., and Honjo, I.: Survivial of patients with cancer of the pancreas in relation to findings on arteriography, Ann. Surg. **179**:37, 1972.
75. Suzuki, T., Kawabe, K., Nakayasu, A., Takeda, H., Kobayashi, K., Kubota, N., and Honjo, I.: Selective arteriography in cancer of the pancreas at a resectable stage, Am. J. Surg. **122**:402, 1971.
76. Uden, R.: Secretin and epinephrine combined in celiac angiography, Acta Radiol. [Diagn.] **17**:17, 1976.
77. Wolfe, W. G., Mullen, D. L., and Silver, D.: Insulinoma of the pancreas, Arch. Surg. **104**:56, 1972.

Ultrasonography

78. Bradley, E. L., and Clements, J. L.: Implications of diagnostic ultrasound in the surgical management of pancreatic pseudocyts, Am. J. Surg. **127**:163, 1974.
79. Doust, B. D., and Pearce, J. D.: Gray scale ultransonic properties of the normal and inflamed pancreas, Radiology **120**:653, 1974.
80. Felson, B., editor: A primer of ultrasound seminars in roentgenology, Radiol. Clin. North Am., vol. 4, no. 4, 1975.
81. Filly, R. A., and Freimanis, A. K.: Echographic diagnosis of pancreatic lesions. Ultrasound scanning techniques and diagnostic findings, Radiology **96**:575, 1970.
82. Fontana, G., Bolondi, L., Conti, M., Plicchi, G., Gullo, L., Caletti, G. C., and Labo, G.: An evaluation of echography in the diagnosis of pancreatic disease, Gut **17**:228, 1976.
83. Hancke, S.: Ultrasonic scanning of the pancreas, J. Clin. Ultrasound **4**:223, 1975.
84. Leopold, G. R.: Pancreatic echography: a new dimension in the diagnosis of pseudocyst, Radiology **104**:365, 1972.
85. Sanders, R. C., editor: Ultrasound, Radiol. Clin. North Am., vol. 13, no. 3, 1975.
86. Weill, F., Kraehenbuhl, J. R., Becker, J. C., Gillet, M., and Bourgoin, A.: Echotomography of the pancreas: a critical and comparative study. In Anacker, H., editor: Efficiency and limits of radiologic examination of the pancreas, Stuttgart, 1975, Georg Thieme, Verlag.

CHAPTER 3

Operative pancreatography

ROBERT E. HERMANN

In 1947 operative pancreatography was introduced and developed by Doubilet and co-workers.[1] They used iodopyracet (Diodrast) injected into the pancreatic duct system by a plastic catheter. The ducts and pancreatic parenchyma were visualized, probably because the iodopyracet was an irritant to the smaller ducts and pancreatic parenchyma. Almost coincidentally with the studies of Doubilet and associates, the French surgeon Leger[3] described a technique of operative pancreatography in 1952. During later studies a water-soluble dye (e.g., 90% Hypaque) was found to be much less irritating and equally effective in visualizing the pancreatic ducts.[2,5-7]

The value of operative pancreatography is that it provides visual identification of the anatomy and pathologic changes of the pancreatic duct system, identifies areas of stenosis and dilatation, and is an important factor in the decision to perform ductal drainage for the treatment of chronic pancreatitis. Operative pancreatography also aids in the identification of pseudocysts of the pancreas and in showing their location and size.[4]

INDICATIONS

Operative pancreatography is indicated in patients with recurrent or chronic pancreatitis to help the surgeon decide whether pancreatic duct drainage or pancreatic resection should be performed. Obviously one might choose to perform solely a drainage operation on a pancreas which shows only evidence of ductal obstruction. Operative pancreatography is also of great value for the patient with a mass in the pancreas suspected of being a pseudocyst because it identifies the size and location of the cyst, helps identify the presence of a multiloculated cyst, and aids in making the decision as to where and how the pseudocyst should be drained.

Operative pancreatography is contraindicated in the patient with acute pancreatitis or subsiding acute inflammation. It should not be performed, or should be performed only with great caution, in the patient whose pancreas appears to be completely normal at operation since there is some risk of inducing inflammatory changes if the pancreatic duct system is overdistended with the instilled dye. The procedure can be performed much more safely in a gland which has undergone previous inflammation and repair with fibrosis of the duct system than in the normal gland unprotected by previous fibrosis.

Interestingly, the pancreatic duct system has been visualized during operative cholangiography in approximately 45% of our patients in whom routine operative cholangiography was performed during biliary surgery. This visualization of the pancreatic duct is usually incomplete since only a small segment of the duct system in the head of the pancreas is seen in most patients. However, in a few patients the entire pancreatic duct system filled with dye and was seen. In some patients pathologic findings of the pancreatic duct system have been unexpectedly encountered (Fig. 3-1).

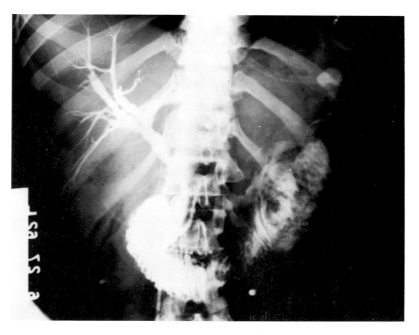

Fig. 3-1. Operative cholangiogram showing the main pancreatic duct. A small pseudocyst is visible in the tail of the pancreas.

TECHNIQUE

The pancreatic duct system can be entered by one of three methods: (1) duodenotomy and transduodenal catheterization of the pancreatic duct through the head of the pancreas, (2) needle aspiration of the midportion of the pancreatic duct system, with instillation of dye into the duct by this means, or (3) amputation of the tail of the pancreas and catheterization of the duct through the distal pancreas (Fig. 3-2).

When a pseudocyst or suspected cystic mass is found in the pancreas, the mass may be aspirated with a needle; and if pancreatic juice or fluid is obtained, about 20 to 30 ml are removed prior to instillation of dye to visualize the cystic cavity (Fig. 3-3).

In the performance of operative pancreatography, it is important not to overfill the pancreatic duct system. Studies by Trapnell and associates[7] have shown that the normal pancreatic duct system accepts approximately 1 ml of dye with visualization of the entire system. When 2 ml of dye are instilled, some of the secondary pancreatic duct tributaries begin to be filled. When more than 2 ml of dye are instilled into a nondilated pancreatic duct system, the secondary and tertiary ducts are uniformly filled and visualized. With the instillation of more than 2 ml of dye, there is also danger of overdistention of the pancreatic duct system, with the hazard of forcing dye into the parenchyma of the gland and potentially activating an episode of pancreatitis. As noted before, this is more likely to occur in a normal gland than in a gland protected by previous fibrosis. An obstructed dilated pancreatic duct system may safely accept from 4 to

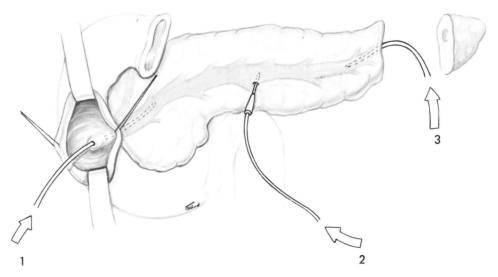

Fig. 3-2. Three methods of operative pancreatography: *1*, transduodenal catheterization of the duct through the papilla of Vater; *2*, mid–pancreatic duct injection; *3*, cannulation of the duct through the distal gland.

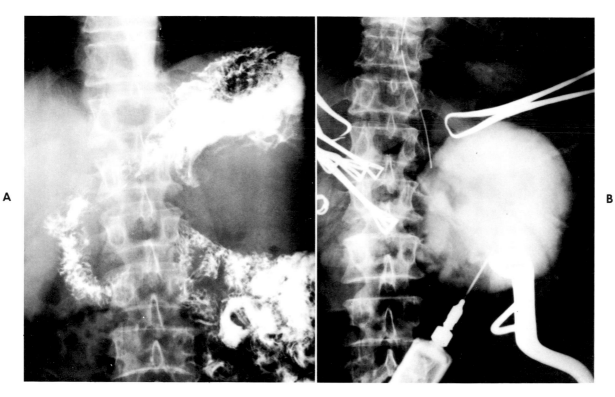

Fig. 3-3. A, Large cystic mass indenting the greater curvature of the stomach. B, Needle aspiration of a pseudocyst in the head of the pancreas has been performed and dye instilled to identify the site and size of the pseudocyst.

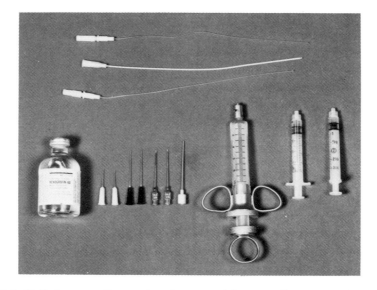

Fig. 3-4. Catheters, needles, and syringes used for operative pancreatography.

10 ml of dye. However, one does not know this unless an initial injection of 2 ml of dye has been given previously.

To prevent overfilling and overdistention of the pancreatic duct system, we use a 2 ml syringe for the initial injection. We select a no. 16 or 18 plastic catheter (Intracath), the largest that can be passed into the pancreatic duct system (Fig. 3-4). The dye we presently use is a water-soluble nonirritating dye, meglumine diatrizoate (Renografin 60). When carefully injected, this dye has proved to be nonirritating to the pancreas and has caused almost no episodes of pancreatitis. After the dye has been instilled and two roentgenograms obtained, it is probably of some importance to aspirate the duct, removing any remaining dye to relieve pressure in the pancreatic duct system.

The decision on which method of pancreatography to use—transduo-

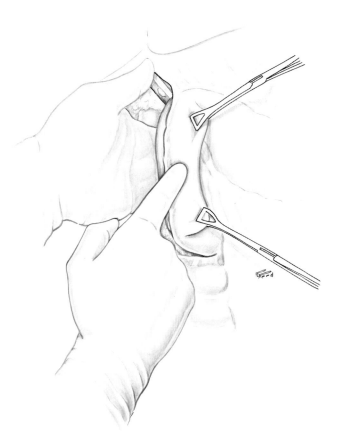

Fig. 3-5. A Kocher maneuver has been performed to mobilize the duodenum from its retroperitoneal position. With the surgeon's left hand behind the duodenum, the right index finger palpates for the papilla of Vater. Localization of the papilla prior to opening the duodenum permits more accurate placement of the duodenotomy incision. If there is difficulty in palpating the papilla, a choledochotomy and passage of a flared French bougie or balloon catheter will facilitate identification of the papilla.

denal, midductal, or distal ductal injection—should be made at surgery. Before any operative pancreatograms are obtained, it is wise to have divided the gastrocolic omentum to expose the entire gland. If the major pathology appears to be in the head of the pancreas or if the entire gland is diseased, then duodenotomy and transduodenal catheterization of the pancreas are indicated (Figs. 3-5 and 3-6).* If these procedures are technically difficult or not possible and the duct is dilated, then another method is preferred. If the pancreatic duct system is dilated and palpable, the easiest way to achieve visualization of this obstructed duct system

*Surgeons who have not had much experience in the direct identification of the papilla of Vater may find it useful to open the common bile duct and pass a small catheter or other suitable instrument through the papilla. A French bougie with a flared end may be used to elevate the papilla into direct view through the open duodenum.

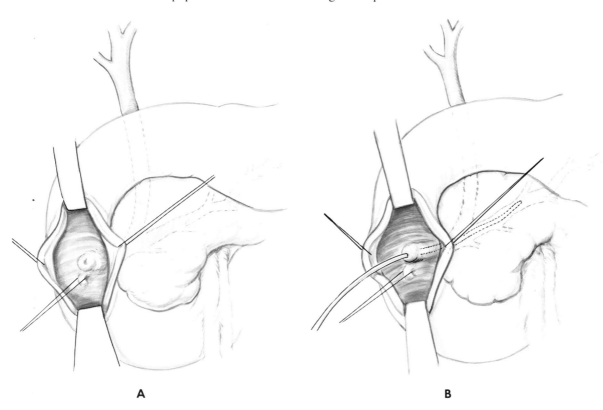

A **B**

Fig. 3-6. A, A longitudinal duodenotomy incision has been made, and the papilla of Vater is seen. Small right angle retractors are placed in the duodenum to aid exposure. A traction suture of 3-0 silk is used below the papilla to bring the medial wall of the duodenum anteriorly and aid in exposure of the papilla. **B,** A no. 18 plastic catheter is passed through the papilla of Vater into the pancreatic duct. This can most often be done without resorting to a sphincterotomy. If the catheter does not pass into the pancreatic duct but goes into the common bile duct, then a sphincterotomy should be performed to enable the surgeon to visualize the pancreatic duct orifice so he can catheterize it directly.

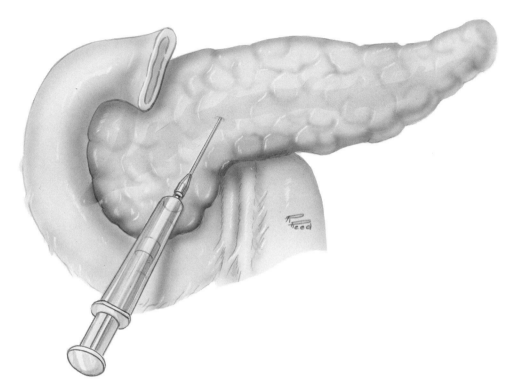

Fig. 3-7. Direct needle injection of the pancreatic duct in its midportion.

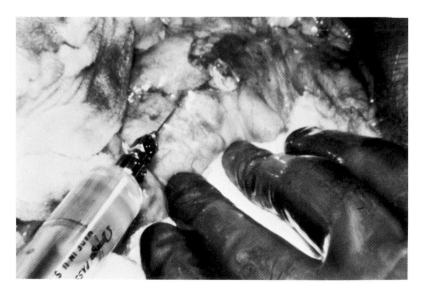

Fig. 3-8. Needle aspiration of the middle pancreatic duct for subsequent injection of dye and an operative pancreatogram.

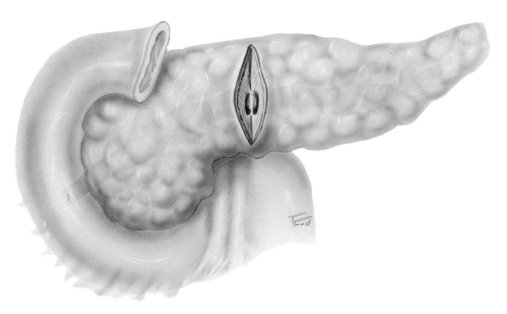

Fig. 3-9. Transverse incision across the middle or distal pancreas to aid in finding the pancreatic duct.

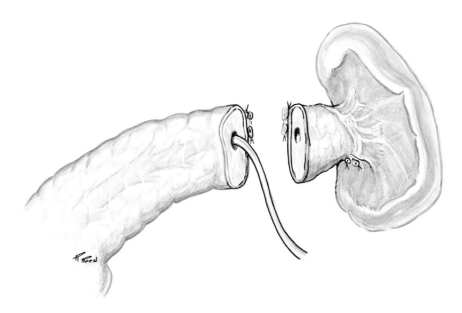

Fig. 3-10. The tail of the pancreas has been amputated along with the spleen. In the proximal divided pancreas the pancreatic duct is located and catheterized for an operative pancreatogram.

may be through a midductal injection of the dilated and palpable pancreatic duct (Figs. 3-7 and 3-8). A no. 18 or 20 needle is selected and the duct is aspirated until 2 to 5 ml of fluid have been removed. Frequently the pancreatic juice found is under pressure. After removal of a moderate amount of pancreatic juice, 2 to 5 ml of meglumine diatrizoate are instilled into the duct for visualization.

Occasionally a midductal injection seems indicated but the duct cannot be palpated and repeated attempts at needle aspiration are unproductive in identifying the location of the pancreatic duct. Then, if the gland is fibrotic, I incise transversely across the upper portion of the pancreas, carefully identifying the location of the splenic vessels to avoid injuring them (Fig. 3-9). The pancreatic duct almost always lies fairly superficially in the upper or cephalad third of the substance of the pancreas, ventral to the splenic vessels. The distal gland will be removed after this study.

If transduodenal catheterization of the pancreatic duct or a midductal injection study is technically difficult or unproductive, the tail of the pancreas is mobilized usually by performing a splenectomy and delivering the distal gland into the operative field along with the splenic vessels. The tail of the pancreas is then amputated and the distal pancreatic duct system is located and entered with a no. 16 or 18 polyethylene catheter (Fig. 3-10). A pancreatogram is then obtained by an injection study through this means.

Operative pancreatograms

Examples of operative pancreatogams which may help the surgeon make his decision for ductal drainage are shown in Figs. 3-11 to 3-16.

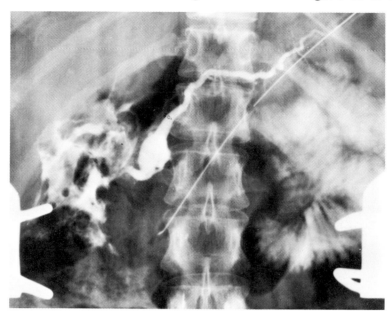

Fig. 3-11. Operative pancreatogram obtained through transduodenal catheterization of the papilla of Vater showing a cystic dilatation of the main pancreatic duct near its opening into the duodenum.

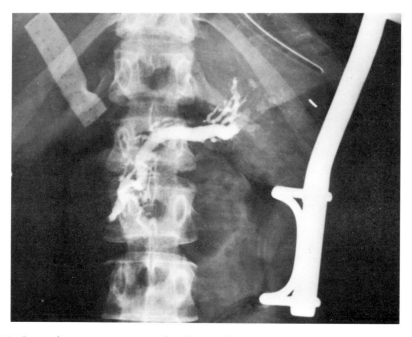

Fig. 3-12. Operative pancreatogram showing a dilated pancreatic duct with stenosis at the papilla of Vater.

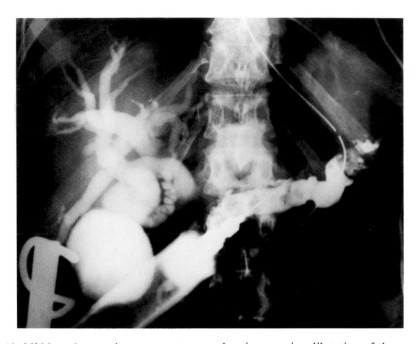

Fig. 3-13. Midductal operative pancreatogram showing massive dilatation of the pancreatic duct. Multiple filling defects (stones) are evident.

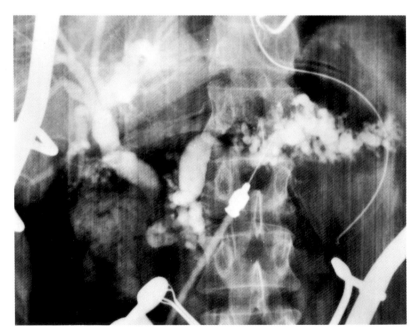

Fig. 3-14. Operative pancreatogram showing multiple areas of stenosis and dilatation (chain-of-lakes deformity) in the distal pancreatic duct system.

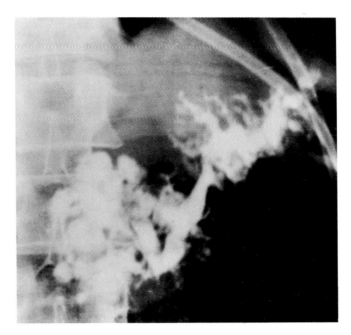

Fig. 3-15. Operative pancreatogram showing a chain-of-lakes deformity and areas of stenosis and dilatation of the entire pancreatic duct system.

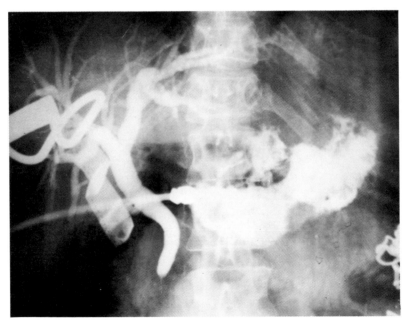

Fig. 3-16. Operative pancreatogram showing a massively dilated pancreatic duct system, almost to the point of pseudocyst formation. An operative cholangiogram done just previously shows a dilated biliary ductal system with no dye passing into the duodenum.

REFERENCES

1. Doubilet, H., Poppel, M. H., and Mulholland, J. H.: Pancreatography; techniques, principles, and observations, Radiology **64:**325, 1955.
2. Howard, J. M., and Short, W. F.: An evaluation of pancreatography in suspected pancreatic disease, Surg. Gynecol. Obstet. **129:**319, 1969.
3. Leger, L.: L'exploration radio-chirurgicale du pancréas et le drainage transpapillaire du canal de Wirsung, J. Chir. **68:**518, 1952.
4. Nardi, G. L., Lyon, D. C., Sheiner, H. J., and Bartlett, M. K.: Solitary occult retention cysts of the pancreas, N. Engl. J. Med. **280:**11, 1969.
5. Rubaum, N. J., and Shohl, T.: X-ray visualization of the pancreas, Ann. Surg. **153:**246, 1961.
6. Thal, A. P., Goott, B., and Margulis, A. R.: Sites of pancreatic duct obstruction in chronic pancreatitis, Ann. Surg. **150:**49, 1959.
7. Trapnell, J. E., Brewster, J., and Howard, J. M.: Transduodenal pancreatography; an improved technique, Surgery **60:**1112, 1966.

CHAPTER 4

Pancreatic biopsy

CALDWELL B. ESSELSTYN, Jr.

Biopsy is a quick, accurate, and safe way to determine the presence or absence of cancer in many anatomic sites; however, this is not the case with ductal carcinoma of the pancreas. Pancreatic biopsy by the Vim-Silverman needle or wedge excision is not safe, is not quick, and is not accurate in the hands of most surgeons and pathologists.

Gambill[5] reported false-negative pancreatic biopsies in 38% of twenty-six patients with documented pancreatic cancer. Coté and co-workers,[3] reporting the Mayo Clinic experience with pancreatic biopsy over several decades, found a high degree of inaccuracy. Wedge resections had false-negative results in 54% of 110 cases, and the Vim-Silverman needle biopsy gave false-negative results in 32% of fifty-three cases. Isaacson and co-workers,[7] reporting more recently on the Mayo Clinic experience, cited a much higher degree of accuracy with the same methods but did not clarify whether this was due to better surgical technique or to improved pathologic evaluation.

Even for the majority of expert surgeons, pancreatic biopsy has proved unreliable. Bowden[2] abandoned pancreatic biopsy in selecting patients for resection because he believed it useless, being false-negative in 27% of thirty-four cases. Probstein and co-workers[10] were equally disenchanted with the accuracy of pancreatic wedge biopsy, finding malignancy in only 43% of twenty-three known cases of pancreatic malignancy. Lightwood and co-workers[9] reporting in 1976, found 17% false-negative reports in eighty-seven cases and an overall mortality of 1.7% and morbidity of 4.7%.

Figures that are more representative of a community experience utilizing biopsy are those of Schultz and Sanders,[11] who collected data on

159 such cases from several Denver hospitals. They found the complication rate of pancreatic fistulas, hemorrhage, infection, and pseudocysts of the pancreas to be 9.5% and the mortality of biopsy alone 3.8%. Especially significant is the mortality; four of the six deaths occurred in patients with benign disease.

The danger and inaccuracy of pancreatic biopsy have led some surgeons to rely on the history, physical examination, laboratory findings, and chiefly the operative findings to determine the diagnosis and operability. Warren and co-workers[15] performed pancreaticoduodenectomy in 218 patients. Six patients had benign disease, an intraoperative false-negative assessment of 3%. This method was far more accurate in the authors' hands than the conventional wedge or needle biopsy.

Perhaps the ultimate testimonial of the difficulty for the pathologist in differentiating the histopathology of the pancreas is the report by Eckert,[4] who performed blind resection in four jaundiced patients with a mass in the head of the pancreas. He was told by the pathologists that all specimens were benign pancreatitis. In follow-up evaluation, all four patients died of recurrent pancreatic cancer in a period of several months to just over five years.

INDIVIDUALIZATION

For most patients with a ductal pancreatic cancer, a biopsy can be performed adjacent to involved nodes (or by excision of an involved node), at the ligament of Treitz, or near the porta hepatis; for others a biopsy of a metastatic liver nodule or a peritoneal implant will confirm the diagnosis (and also the incurability of the lesion). Without any sign of overt spread or with disease apparently limited to the pancreas, the newer experience with fine needle biopsy[1,8] has proved to be safe and accurate (Fig. 4-1, *A*). There have been no deaths or serious complications, and in more than 70% of the cases this method has been accurate. It has replaced other biopsy methods at our hospital.

Since islet cell tumors are more demarcated without the scirrhous reaction of ductal carcinoma and rarely cause jaundice, a small shaving-type biopsy (Fig. 4-1, *B*) of the surface of these tumors is diagnostic and useful for resectable lesions. Because the same is true for the rare cystadenocarcinoma, which is conspicuous by its gross cystic enlargement, the diagnosis is confirmed by biopsy of the cyst wall. A shaving biopsy may also be done for adenocarcinoma that has grossly penetrated the pancreatic capsule.

Results of recent studies[6,13,14] have shown a high degree of accuracy and safety with computed tomography–guided percutaneous biopsy in patients with mass pancreatic lesions. In poor-risk patients with advanced disease,

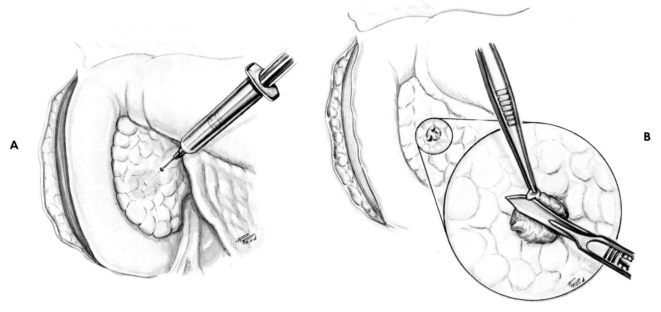

Fig. 4-1. A, Direct fine needle (no. 23 gauge) aspiration biopsy of pancreatic cancer. The aspirate is placed on a glass slide, fixed, and then read. **B,** Direct shave biopsy of a protruding pancreatic cancer that has penetrated the anterior surface.

the need for laparotomy is eliminated. For others time at exploration is saved. (See Chapter 2.)

For ampullary lesions a diagnosis may be obtained preoperatively by endoscopic biopsy—permitting a safe, accurate, and noncontaminating biopsy.

For lesions of the head of the pancreas that cannot be differentiated from the more favorable duodenal or distal common bile duct lesions, several other options are available:

1. The endoscope may be passed at surgery and precisely guided intra-abdominally by the surgeon, permitting the endoscopist to obtain biopsy specimens which the pathologists may differentiate from pancreatic cancer.[12]

2. In other situations a hard spicule or "horn" of neoplastic tissue may be found beyond the duodenal serosa or pancreatic capsule that will permit a safe "shave" of the lesion (Fig. 4-1, *B*)

3. If indecision persists despite these maneuvers, in cases that may or may not be pancreatic carcinoma, the surgeon can fully mobilize the lesion and evaluate its operability. At this point we would obtain an intraoperative and "scrubbed-up" consultation with a second and often a third senior surgeon. If consensus favors a lesion with hope for cure in a patient who is young and of adequate physiologic reserve, a resection is performed.

Therefore I endorse pancreatic resection under these circumstances even though definitive preoperative diagnosis has not been made.

REFERENCES

1. Arnejo, B., Stormby, N., and Akerman, M.: Cytodiagnosis of pancreatic lesions by means of fine-needle biopsy during operation, Acta Chir. Scand. **138:**363, 1972.
2. Bowden, L.: The fallibility of pancreatic biopsy, Ann. Surg. **139:**403, 1954.
3. Coté, J., Dockerty, M. B., and Priestley, J. T.: An evaluation of pancreatic biopsy with the Vim-Silverman needle, Arch. Surg. **79:**588, 1959.
4. Eckert, C.: Personal communication, June, 1976.
5. Gambill, E. E.: Pancreatitis associated with pancreatic carcinoma; a study of 26 cases, Mayo Clin. Proc. **46:**174, 1971.
6. Hancke, S., Holm, H., and Koch, F.: Ultrasonically guided percutaneous fine needle biopsy of the pancreas, Surg. Gynecol. Obstet. **140:**361, 1975.
7. Isaacson, R., Weiland, L. H., and McIlrath, D. C.: Biopsy of the pancreas, Arch. Surg. **109:**227, 1974.
8. Koivuniemi, A., Lempinen, M., and Pantzar, P.: Fine needle aspiration biopsy of pancreas, Ann. Chir. Gynaecol. Fenn. **61:**273, 1972.
9. Lightwood, R., Reber, H. A., and Way, L. W.: The risk and accuracy of pancreatic biopsy, Am. J. Surg. **132:**189, 1976.
10. Probstein, J. G., Sachar, L., and Rindskoph, W.: Biopsies of pancreatic masses, Surgery **27:**356, 1950.
11. Schultz, N. J., and Sanders, R. J.: Evaluation of pancreatic biopsy, Ann. Surg. **158:**1053, 1963.
12. Sivak, M. V., Jr., Esselstyn, C. B., Jr., and Owens, F. J.: Intraoperative upper gastrointestinal endoscopy and biopsy; case report, Cleve. Clin. Q. **41:**67, 1974.
13. Smith, E. H., Bartru, R. J., Jr., Chang, Y. C., D'Orsi, C. J., Lokich, J., Abbruzzese, A., and Dantono, J.: Percutaneous aspiration biopsy of the pancreas under ultrasonic guidance, N. Engl. J. Med. **292:**825, 1975.
14. Tylén, U., Arnesjo, B., Lindberg, L. G., Lunderquist, A., and Akerman, M.: Percutaneous biopsy of carcinoma of pancreas guided by angiography. Surg. Gynecol. Obstet. **142:**737, 1976.
15. Warren, K. W., Cattell, R. B., Blackburn, J. P., and Nora, P. F.: A long-term appraisal of pancreaticoduodenal resection for periampullary carcinoma, Ann. Surg. **155:**653, 1962.

CHAPTER 5

Acute pancreatitis

AVRAM M. COOPERMAN

The role of surgery in acute pancreatitis remains limited and controversial. The three most common conditions associated with pancreatitis are biliary disease, alcohol, and postoperative states (usually following biliary and gastric surgery).[20] Even though cholelithiasis and alcohol (the latter possibly having a direct toxic effect on the pancreas[14]) are commonly associated with acute pancreatitis, the cause of the pancreatitis remains unknown.

Several recent reviews have summarized the etiology and pathophysiology of acute pancreatitis.[1,5,11,20] Whatever the cause of the disease, pancreatic secretions gain access to the interstitium of the gland and there incite a spectrum of catalytic and autodigestive enzymatic changes.

Early interstitial change is characterized by interacinar edema (with minimal hemorrhage), and this disease is acute edematous pancreatitis. Whatever the cause, edematous pancreatitis tends to be benign and self-limited in 80% of cases.[11,19] Therefore it is difficult to know what specific treatment should be used and how treatment alters the course of the disease.[15]

In a small group of patients (perhaps 10% to 20%), the disease progresses to or begins as a more fulminant and aggressive process—which has been called acute necrotizing or hemorrhagic pancreatitis—with mortality up to 90%.[9,13,18] The reasons why edematous pancreatitis may progress to or begin in this form remain unclear. Indirect evidence suggests that in many instances hemorrhagic and edematous pancreatitis are related and that edematous pancreatitis commonly precedes hemorrhagic pancreatitis.[11]

Although the diagnosis of hemorrhagic pancreatitis may be apparent in most instances, the diagnosis is made with more difficulty in postoperative patients. Unexplained shock (due to hypovolemia) and/or severe abdominal pain (and elevated serum amylase levels) are clues to this diagnosis and may be presenting symptoms.

Since the mortality rate is high in hemorrhagic pancreatitis, it would be desirable if these patients could be identified early in the course of an attack so a more aggressive treatment might be considered in selected instances. Ranson and co-workers[13] evaluated 100 cases of acute pancreatitis (most were alcoholics) to identify a high-risk group. Eleven factors were found to correlate with increased morbidity and mortality—including age (over 55 years), a white blood cell count greater than 16,000 per cubic millimeter, a blood glucose value greater than 200 mg per deciliter, a serum glutamic-oxalacetic transaminase (SGOT) greater than 225 IU, and an elevated blood urea nitrogen (BUN). When three or more factors were present, 62% of patients died and an additional 33% were seriously ill.

If the prognostic importance of three or more of these factors is confirmed by other surgeons, then an accurate prediction of morbidity and mortality will be available.* These high-risk patients are usually identified within the first 48 hours of hospitalization because they fail to respond to usual treatment or they deteriorate. In this small group several alternatives have been suggested:

1. Peritoneal lavage (without laparotomy)[2,13,14,16]
2. Laparotomy with insertion of drains into the lesser sac with or without gastrostomy, cholecystostomy, or jejunostomy[6,13,18,19]
3. Major pancreatic resection[4,7,8,10,12,13,21]

For several reasons it has been difficult to evaluate and compare the practical and theoretical merits of each of these methods: the number of patients has been few, the causes of the pancreatitis have been different, the patient population has been dissimilar, and the criteria for surgery have been variable. These factors coupled with our lack of basic knowledge of the disease processes limit significant analysis of data.

PERITONEAL LAVAGE (Fig. 5-1)

The use of peritoneal lavage for pancreatitis was described forty years ago[17] but did not receive clinical attention until Rodgers and Carey[14] showed a beneficial effect in dogs. The canine pancreas is intraperitoneal. Whether the results are applicable in man, in whom the pancreas is retro-

---

*Recently Jacobs and co-workers[8] analyzed 519 cases of acute pancreatitis. The overall mortality rate was 12.9%. Shock requiring massive colloid replacement, hypocalcemia, and renal and respiratory failure were associated with a high nonoperative mortality rate (70%).

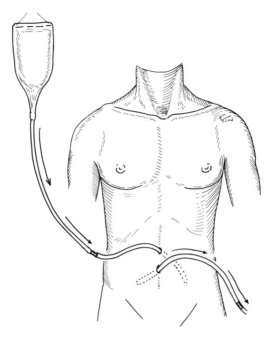

Fig. 5-1. Sump drains are placed in the lower midline by a cutdown on the abdominal wall or by dialysis trochar catheters. Continuous lavage with isotonic solutions is begun. The short incisions are midline and infraumbilical.

peritoneal, is unclear. Certainly a beneficial effect has followed the percutaneous placement and irrigation of catheters into the peritoneal cavity in many patients.[2,13] These positive effects have been attributed to dilution of toxic or vasoactive substances dialyzed through an inflamed retroperitoneal surface or dialysis of toxic substances through the bloodstream. Since this procedure can be instituted at the bedside, it is appealing from a simple as well as a practical standpoint. I use this treatment early in deteriorating patients or in those with poor prognostic signs even though its value is unproved.

SUMP DRAINAGE (Fig. 5-2)

Placement of sump drains by operative means into the lesser sac was advocated by Waterman and co-workers.[19] The basis of this work was first experimental and then clinical. Nine of ten patients with hemorrhagic pancreatitis improved. It was postulated that drainage of exudate or peripancreatic secretions alters the course of disease by limiting absorption of vasoactive and toxic substances. It would be interesting if publications on this method quantitated the amount of drainage which followed placement of these sumps or reported on the nature of the drainage. I have not utilized this method by itself.

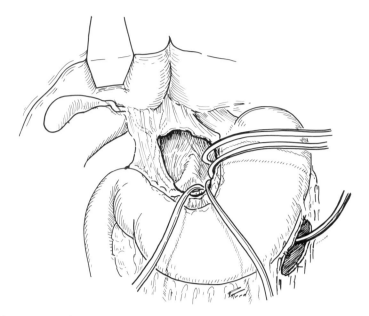

Fig. 5-2. If laparotomy is performed, one should open the lesser sac on both curvatures of the stomach and insert drainage catheters. The gallbladder may be decompressed by a Foley catheter. I prefer to do an operative cholangiogram; if there is no biliary obstruction, I do not decompress the biliary tree. If the stomach is obstructed by an inflammatory mass, a gastrojejunal bypass is needed. If there is no obstruction, a nasogastric tube is sufficient.

SUMP DRAINAGE AND MULTIPLE OSTOMIES

Besides sump drainage—cholecystostomy, gastrostomy, and feeding jejunostomy in hemorrhagic pancreatitis have been used by some surgeons to improve survival. These additions may have a beneficial effect on the course of hemorrhagic pancreatitis by decompressing the gastric and biliary tree and allowing tube feedings via the jejunum. In one series an anticipated mortality of 90% was reduced to 34% (thirteen of thirty-eight patients).[18]

The need for two or all three of these procedures has been questioned. If gallstones are not present and the common duct is not obstructed (it will not be in up to 80% of patients), then little would be gained from decompressing the biliary tree. Jejunostomy feedings are well tolerated, but parenteral nutrition may be as good as if not better than this.[21] An alternate route to jejunostomy feedings may be via a Hurwitz tube used as both a gastrostomy for drainage and a jejunostomy for feeding. Finally, since the need for a gastrostomy is predicated on prolonged ileus or gastric retention, it may prove to be unnecessary in a substantial number of patients.

PANCREATIC RESECTION (Fig. 5-3)

Although a direct surgical approach on the pancreas seems hazardous, there have been many reports of pancreatic resections of various degrees in selected deteriorating patients with hemorrhagic pancreatitis. In 1970 Hollender and co-workers[7] reported on thirteen patients who underwent 95% pancreatectomy for fulminating hemorrhagic pancreatitis. Norton and Eiseman[12] have reported on four patients who underwent pancreatic resection; three survived. I have had two experiences with this procedure; one patient survived. A resected specimen is shown in Fig. 5-4.

Ranson and co-workers[13] assessed prospectively sump drainage, gastrostomy, cholecystostomy, and jejunostomy versus conservative treatment (nonoperative) in a few patients with hemorrhagic pancreatitis. Although the number of patients was few (ten) and the mortality rate

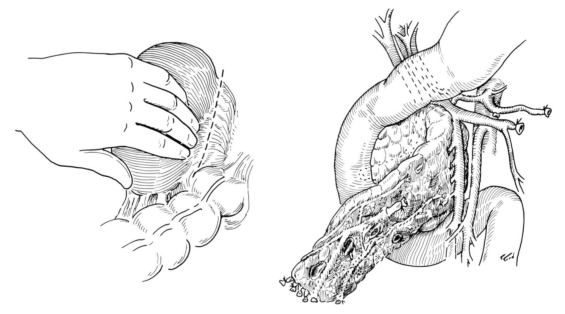

Fig. 5-3. If pancreatectomy is to be done for hemorrhagic pancreatitis, the technique is similar to distal pancreatic resection. There are a number of guidelines. (1) In deteriorating patients the operation should be done within 72 hours of onset of an attack. The planes of dissection are not difficult to see at this time. (2) The key to the operation is preliminary posterolateral mobilization of the spleen and pancreas. This will expose the tail of the pancreas, and the dissection is posterior to the pancreas (which is relatively free of reaction). (3) Most of the dissection can be done manually. Small vessels frequently are thrombosed by pancreatitis. Since it is difficult to know where viable pancreas is, I dissect to the mesenteric vessels and divide the gland at that point. (4) The pathologist then examines the gland to see whether normal pancreas is present at this level. If the gland is not satisfactory, the dissection may be carried to the right of the mensenteric vessels; but I do not dissect beyond this point in critically ill patients. Drains are placed to the transected gland.

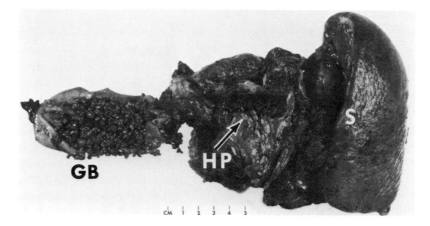

Fig. 5-4. Operative specimen of acute hemorrhagic pancreatitis. The spleen *(S)*, resected pancreas with hemorrhagic pancreatitis *(HP)*, and gallbladder with multiple stones *(GB)* are shown. This patient died 4 days postoperatively of progressive pulmonary insufficiency.

similar, a higher incidence of pulmonary complications and intra-abdominal sepsis followed surgical treatment. These patients had alcoholic pancreatitis. Five other patients underwent pancreatic resection, and all died. Because of the high mortality rate associated with each of the procedures, there remains good argument for the early nonoperative approach when possible.

The use of parenteral nutrition and later surgery for the complications of pancreatitis (abscess, pseudocyst) is gaining support.[21] This presupposes that the patient will survive the initial period of pancreatitis, which is evidently not so in many series.

Finally, an alternate ingenious approach has been suggested by Brzek and Bartoš,[3] who cannulated the thoracic duct in the neck and noted a decrease in toxicity and improvement in survival. It has been shown that pancreatic and peripancreatic fluid is absorbed and transported by the lymphatics and then into the bloodstream. This method is unproved and has had limited clinical application.

PERSONAL OBSERVATION

It is difficult to individualize treatment and decisions for a patient with necrotizing pancreatitis. In my practice patients with three or more poor prognostic signs (as defined by Ranson and co-workers[13]) are initially monitored by Swan-Ganz catheter and blood gases. Early peritoneal lavage is done by percutaneous catheter placement. If the patient deteriorates despite these measures (fluid replacement, respiratory care), I consider exploration. If the biliary tree is not obstructed and hemorrhagic pancreatitis is found, the decision is between (1) placing sump drains in the lesser sac and (2) resecting the gland. My inclination at present, based on a relatively healthy usually nonalcoholic group of patients, is to resect (from tail to body) to viable pancreas (or to the uncinate process). Early in the course of the disease, this can be done quickly without much difficulty. My opinion is subject to change, however, as more data become available.

REFERENCES

1. Barraclough, B. H., and Coupland, G. A. E.: Acute pancreatitis: a review, Aust. N. Z. J. Surg. **41**:211, 1972.
2. Bolooki, H., and Gliedman, M. L.: Peritoneal dialysis in treatment of acute pancreatitis, Surgery **64**:466, 1968.
3. Brzek, V., and Bartoš, V.: Therapeutic effect of the prolonged thoracic duct lymph fistula in patients with acute pancreatitis, Digestion **2**:43, 1969.
4. Dritsas, K. G.: Near total pancreatectomy in the treatment of acute hemorrhagic pancreatitis, Am. J. Surg. **42**:44, 1976.
5. Feller, J. H., Brown, R. A., Toussaint, G. P., and Thompson, A. G.: Changing methods in the treatment of severe pancreatitis, Am. J. Surg. **127**:196, 1974.
6. Fock, G., and Kyosola, K.: Conservative surgery in acute pancreatitis, Ann. Chir. Gynaecol. Fenn. **64**:88, 1975.
7. Hollender, L. F., Gillet, M., and Sava, G.: La pancréatectomie d'urgence dans les pancréatites aigues. A propos de 13 observations, Ann. Chir. **24**:647, 1970.
8. Jacobs, M., Daggett, W. M., Civetta, J. M., Vasu, M. A., Lawson, D. W., Warshaw, A. L., Nardi, G. L., and Bartlett, M. K.: Acute pancreatitis: analysis of factors influencing survival, Ann. Surg. **185**:43, 1977.
9. Jordan, G. L., and Spjut, H. J.: Hemorrhagic pancreatitis, Arch. Surg. **104**:489, 1972.
10. Khedroo, L. G., and Casella, P. A.: Acute hemorrhagic pancreatitis; beneficial effects of primary excision of grossly necrotic pancreatic tissue, Ill. Med. J. **129**:61, 1966.
11. Knight, M. J., and Ballinger, W. F.: Pathophysiology, progression, and treatment of acute pancreatitis. In Ballinger, W. F., and Drapanas, T., editors: Practice of surgery: current review, vol. 2, St. Louis, 1975, The C. V. Mosby Co.
12. Norton, L., and Eiseman, B.: Near total pancreatectomy for hemorrhagic pancreatitis, Am. J. Surg. **127**:191, 1974.
13. Ranson, J. H. C., Rifkind, K. M., Roses, D. F., Fink, S. D., Eng. K., and Spencer, F. C.: Prognostic signs and the role of operative management in acute pancreatitis, Surg. Gynecol. Obstet. **139**:69, 1974.
14. Rodgers, R. E., and Carey, L. C.: Peritoneal lavage in experimental pancreatitis in dogs, Am. J. Surg. **111**:792, 1966.
15. Schapiro, H., Wruble, L. D., and Britt, L. G.: The possible mechanism of alcohol in the production of acute pancreatitis, Surgery **60**:1108, 1966.
16. Trapnell, J. E.: Natural history and prognosis of acute pancreatitis, Ann. R. Coll. Surg. Engl. **38**:265, 1966.
17. Wakeley, C. P. G., and Hunter, J. B.: In Rose, W., and Carless, A., editors: Manual of surgery, vol. 2, ed. 15, London, 1937, Balliere, Tindall & Cassell, Ltd.
18. Warshaw, A. L., Imbembo, A. L., Civetta, J. M., and Daggett, W. M.: Surgical intervention in acute necrotizing pancreatitis, Am. J. Surg. **127**:484, 1974.
19. Waterman, N. G., Walsky, R., Kasdan, M. L., and Abrams, B. L.: The treatment of acute hemorrhagic pancreatitis by sump drainage, Surg. Gynecol. Obstet. **126**:963, 1968.
20. White, T. T.: Inflammatory diseases of the pancreas, Adv. Surg. **9**:247, 1975.
21. White, T. T., and Heimbach, D. M.: Sequestrectomy and hyperalimentation in the treatment of hemorrhagic pancreatitis, Am. J. Surg. **132**:270, 1976.

CHAPTER 6

Pseudocysts

AVRAM M. COOPERMAN
STANLEY O. HOERR

Pseudocysts of the pancreas are cystic accumulations of fluid rich in enzymes. They infrequently develop after pancreatitis, carcinoma, or trauma and presumably arise from collections of pancreatic secretions that may follow ductal disruption, acinar injury, or both. They are differentiated from true cystic lesions of the pancreas by the absence of a glandular epithelial lining.[6,36]

INCIDENCE

The frequency and incidence of pseudocysts developing after trauma are unknown. The incidence in chronic pancreatitis is 2% to 10%.[17,29,31,33] The incidence after severe acute pancreatitis may be as high as 50% when sonography is used for diagnosis.[6] Of 100 cystic lesions of the pancreas, eighty to ninety will be pseudocysts and ten cystadenomas or cystadenocarcinomas.[26]

DIAGNOSIS

Regardless of etiology, the presenting symptoms and signs are similar. Epigastric pain or fullness, anorexia, and weight loss are the most common symptoms.[26,29] In one third to one half of patients, the pseudocyst is palpable and detected by the patient as well as by the examiner.[34] A recent history of trauma or pancreatitis accompanies these findings in most patients. In 10% of patients, atypical features or location of presentation exist—including jaundice, gastrointestinal hemorrhage, pancreatic ascites, and intrasplenic, cervical, and mediastinal presentations.*

*References 3, 8, 11, 14, 15, 22, 28, 32, 38.

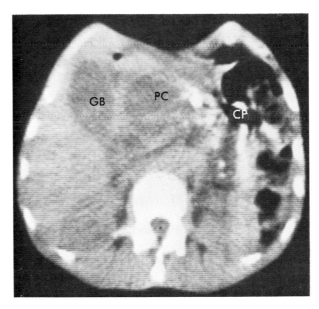

Fig. 6-1. Computed tomographic scan of the upper abdomen showing a large pseudocyst *(PC)*, a dilated gallbladder and cystic duct *(GB)*, and calcific pancreatitis *(CP)*.

In all patients suspected of having a pancreatic pseudocyst, routine laboratory tests are obtained. Elevations in serum and urine amylase are the most common laboratory abnormalities (seen in two thirds of patients).[33]

A plain roentgenogram of the abdomen is taken. A homogeneous density may suggest a mass in the region of the lesser sac. Widening of the duodenal loop and displacement of the gastric bubble or transverse colon are findings suggestive of a lesser sac mass. Liquid calcifications in the pseudocyst may rarely be seen.[35] Barium examination of the stomach and upper intestine may reveal widening of the duodenal loop or displacement or compression of the stomach. Barium studies of the colon may show downward displacement of the left transverse colon. The results of these tests are helpful in up to 90% of patients. An echogram or computed tomographic scan may localize the cystic area and indicate whether the mass is solid or cystic (Fig. 6-1).[18]

UNUSUAL MANIFESTATIONS

The presence of jaundice with pancreatic pseudocysts may imply either compression of the common bile duct by a pseudocyst located in the head of the pancreas or intrapancreatic obstruction of the distal common bile duct by chronic pancreatitis.[10,19,31] A carcinoma obstructing the pancreatic duct is an infrequent but important associated factor with pseudocysts. This should be considered in recurrent pseudocysts or when the history is not compatible with pancreatitis or trauma.

TREATMENT

The decision whom to treat and when and how to treat a patient with a pancreatic pseudocyst must be based on the natural history of the disease and the potential risks and benefits of surgery. There is limited information on the natural history of pseudocysts. The major reason for this lack is that the exact incidence is not known. Recently echograms and other scans have been used as routine diagnostic tests in pancreatitis and abdominal trauma. Many small cystic lesions previously unrecognized may have resolved spontaneously; they now can be diagnosed and followed.[4-6] Larger and symptomatic pseudocysts have obviously formed the basis of most published reports. Bradley and co-workers[6] used echography to follow ninety-two patients with moderately severe acute pancreatitis. Fluid collections in the lesser sac developed in fifty-two patients.

Two methods of treatment of pancreatic pseudocysts are available: observation and surgery.

Observation

Some pseudocysts spontaneously regress—presumably by resorption of fluid through the cyst wall, drainage through a major pancreatic duct system, or rupture into an adjacent viscus.[6] Bradley and Clements[4] initially showed by serial echograms that spontaneous resolution of acute pseudocysts does occur. Their most recent report stated that one fourth of acute pseudocysts resolved spontaneously, usually within 6 weeks after detection.[6] Which pseudocysts will resolve is unpredictable, but this information will hopefully be derived from additional prospective studies. At present, small (less than 5 cm) asymptomatic pseudocysts can be followed after an echogram for 2 to 3 months before surgery is contemplated.[4-6]

Besides possible spontaneous regression of the pseudocyst, another factor which favors observation is the uncertainty whether a given mass is truly cystic rather than inflammatory. More than one abdominal exploration has been done for a presumed pseudocyst and a large inflammatory phlegmon (pseudopseudocyst) has been found.[16,30] This again emphasizes the importance of a positive preoperative echogram or scan.

Arguments against observing pseudocysts are based on the potential complications that can occur—including perforation,[2,10] hemorrhage[8,12,14,20] and infection.[25] The incidence of these complications is unknown and may be overemphasized. It is likely that complications of pseudocysts are more apt to be reported than uncomplicated pseudocysts.

Hemorrhage from a pancreatic pseudocyst is not a frequent occurrence. It may develop from the cyst wall or, more commonly, may be caused by erosion of the pseudocyst into a major artery or vein (usually the splenic).* In these patients preoperative arteriography can be helpful

*References 8, 12, 13, 14, 20.

to both localize the bleeding site and perhaps control bleeding by pressor infusion. In 1967 Cogbill[12] reported two cases of hemorrhage associated with pseudocysts and reviewed fourteen other reported cases. Eleven of these occurred after surgical drainage. A mortality of 50% with a hemorrhagic pseudocyst may have reflected unaggressive and often inaccurate therapy and may also reflect extensive inflammation of the surrounding pancreas. Today this mortality should be less with earlier, more accurate, and aggressive therapy.

In general, ligation of the splenic artery with or without splenectomy plus drainage of the pseudocyst will control the hemorrhage and decompress the pseudocyst. Free perforation with intraperitoneal leakage of a pseudocyst occurs in less than 5% of patients.[21] The recorded instances of free perforation are sufficiently few that the size, cause, and duration of the pseudocysts have not permitted characterization. Such a complication is more likely to occur in acute pseudocysts with friable immature walls. In these instances external drainage with a catheter will control or prevent free perforation.

Surgical treatment

Usually a detectable pseudocyst that does not resolve will require drainage or excision. Although percutaneous aspiration was first attempted by Lucke and Klebs in 1867,[24] it ended fatally. Perhaps aspirations guided by echography or endoscopy will be future ways to drain pseudocysts. These methods have not been widely attempted, however.

Timing of operation. The optimal time to drain a pseudocyst would ideally be when it is most mature and has not yet caused complications. Although the time interval is not known, some experimental evidence has indicated that 6 weeks are necessary for the pseudocyst wall to thicken sufficiently to allow internal drainage to be done.[9,27]

This delay may be questioned, but a retrospective review of pseudocysts by Cerilli and Faris[9] showed much higher mortality and morbidity rates when pseudocysts were drained internally before 6 weeks.

Principles of surgery. The principles of operative treatment of pancreatic pseudocysts have been emphasized by Warren and co-workers.[36]
1. No single operation is suitable for treatment of all these cysts.
2. The choice must be individualized to the nature of the cyst and the condition of the patient.
3. The initial operation may be temporizing and lifesaving.
4. Internal or external drainage should be done only when the presence of neoplasia has been ruled out.

Operations. The available operations are
1. External drainage
2. Internal drainage
3. Excision of the pseudocyst

External drainage. External drainage of pseudocysts is used when acute pseudocysts with thin walls require drainage or when an infected pseudocyst is encountered. In a collected series 25% of pseudocysts were so treated.[29] This treatment is necessary because of infection in the cyst, peritonitis, or rapid increase in size with obstruction of a nearby viscus. Three routes of infection have been suggested: transcolonic, hematogenous, or peroral.

External drainage (by a percutaneous technique) was first employed in 1867,[24] but the patient died of peritonitis in the early postoperative period. After external drainage, pancreatic fistulas develop in 25% of patients and may require subsequent surgery.[29] However, fistulas do not develop in three fourths of patients. Whether these are the patients whose pseudocyst communicates with a major duct system is not known.

Internal drainage. Internal drainage is the most popular means of decompressing pancreatic pseudocysts today. Jedlicka,[23] in 1921, first described cystogastrostomy. By leaving a catheter in the cyst and doing contrast studies, he noted that the size of the cyst cavity was reduced by half in 7 days and was obliterated in 14 to 21 days.

Although stomach, duodenum, and small intestine are commonly used to join the pseudocyst, the organ of choice is the one adherent to the cyst wall. This means that all will be used at varying times. In one large review of pseudocysts, cystogastrostomy was done in 45%, cystoduodenostomy in 16%, cystojejunostomy in 8%, and excision of the pseudocyst in 4%.[2]

At the time of surgery but before draining a pseudocyst, we have advocated getting a pseudocystogram (Fig. 6-2). After a small amount of fluid has been aspirated from the pseudocyst and an injection of water-soluble contrast material (Renografin) made, a roentgenogram is taken. This will demonstrate whether the pseudocyst communicates with the main pancreatic duct or is multiloculated. Although the former situation is of academic interest, the latter is of practical importance because a larger opening to an adjoining pseudocyst cavity may be required to provide effective drainage. Whatever anastomosis is employed, a biopsy of the wall of the pseudocyst should be performed to exclude a neoplastic cyst. A neoplasm may be present in a benign-appearing cyst lacking inflammatory adhesions.

Of interest is the fate of the pseudocyst when internal drainage has been effected. Further studies (comprising three patients) have confirmed Jedlicka's early observation.[7] The pseudocyst wall collapses between 1 and 3 weeks after internal drainage.[7] Endoscopic examination of a cystogastrostomy anastomosis shows obliteration of the anastomosis by 1 week. Early fears that barium or food would reflux from the stomach or duodenum into the pseudocyst generally have not been substantiated and

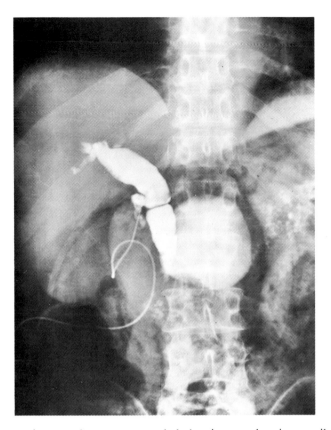

Fig. 6-2. Intraoperative pseudocystogram and cholangiogram showing a unilocular pseudocyst and an obstructed distal common bile duct. The cause of this was chronic pancreatitis, and a Roux-en-Y cystojejunostomy and side-to-side choledochojejunostomy was done.

probably reflect the normal peristaltic and motility pattern of the stomach and duodenum.

Excision of the pseudocyst. The pseudocyst is excised in less than 10% of cases.[22,34,36] This operation may be done when the pseudocyst is confined to the tail of the pancreas. We have not performed this operation for pseudocysts but have preferred internal drainage, which is an easier operation with less morbidity.

RECURRENCE

It is difficult to state whether recurrent pseudocysts are, in fact, recurrent newly formed second pseudocysts or residual and incompletely drained primary lesions.

Thus "recurrent" in most reviews must be interpreted to mean that persistent or *new* pseudocysts develop in 10% of patients.[2] This percentage is not surprising and may reflect a subsequent complication of pancreatitis in some alcoholic patients.

Surgical techniques

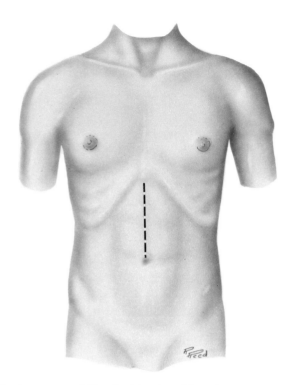

Fig. 6-3. An upper midline incision is utilized in nearly all cases.

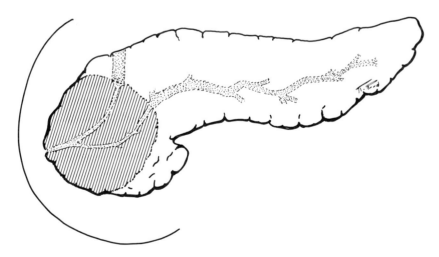

Fig. 6-4. Pseudocyst in the head of the pancreas with partial obstruction of the pancreatic duct and common bile duct.

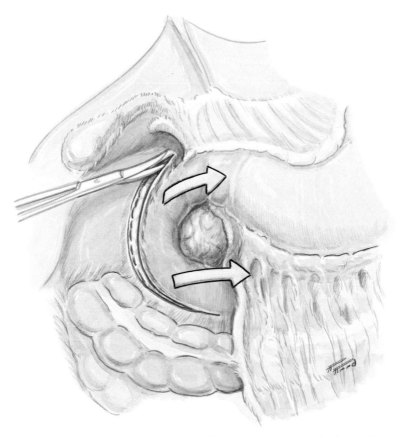

Fig. 6-5. The lateral peritoneal attachments of the duodenum are incised (Kocher maneuver) and the duodenum mobilized. Freeing the duodenum from the surrounding retroperitoneal structures facilitates bimanual palpation of the head of the gland.

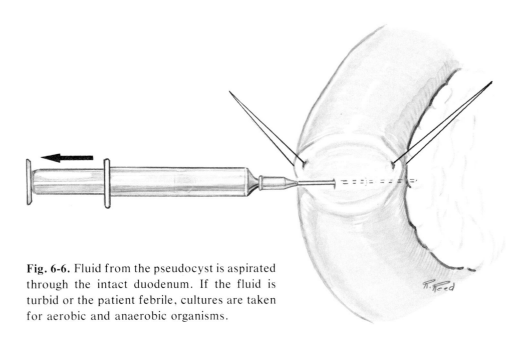

Fig. 6-6. Fluid from the pseudocyst is aspirated through the intact duodenum. If the fluid is turbid or the patient febrile, cultures are taken for aerobic and anaerobic organisms.

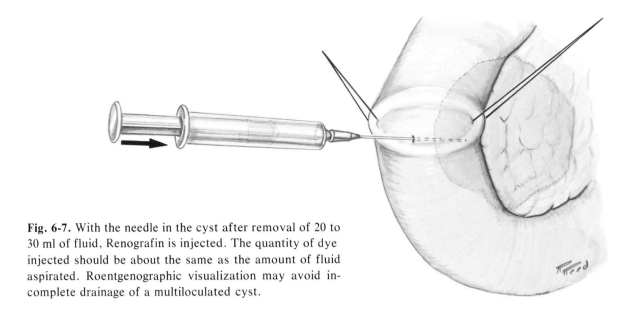

Fig. 6-7. With the needle in the cyst after removal of 20 to 30 ml of fluid, Renografin is injected. The quantity of dye injected should be about the same as the amount of fluid aspirated. Roentgenographic visualization may avoid incomplete drainage of a multiloculated cyst.

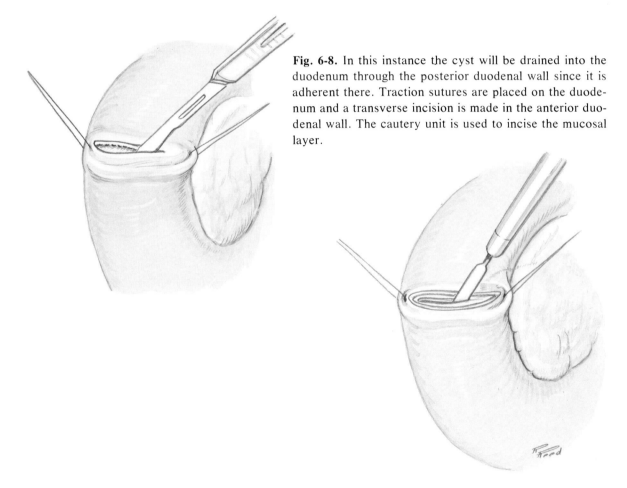

Fig. 6-8. In this instance the cyst will be drained into the duodenum through the posterior duodenal wall since it is adherent there. Traction sutures are placed on the duodenum and a transverse incision is made in the anterior duodenal wall. The cautery unit is used to incise the mucosal layer.

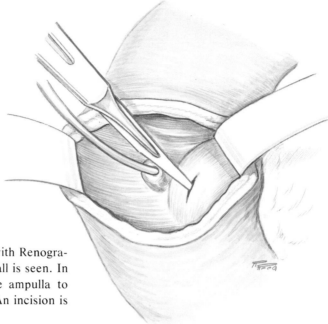

Fig. 6-9. When the cyst has been distended with Renografin, an impression on the medial duodenal wall is seen. In this case a fine probe was passed into the ampulla to protect the pancreatic duct during surgery. An incision is made into the pseudocyst with a scalpel.

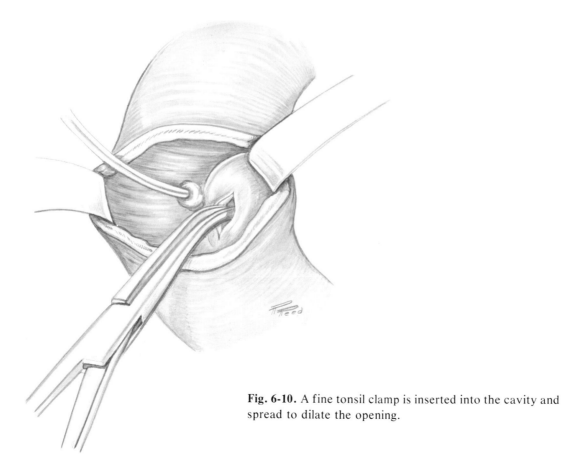

Fig. 6-10. A fine tonsil clamp is inserted into the cavity and spread to dilate the opening.

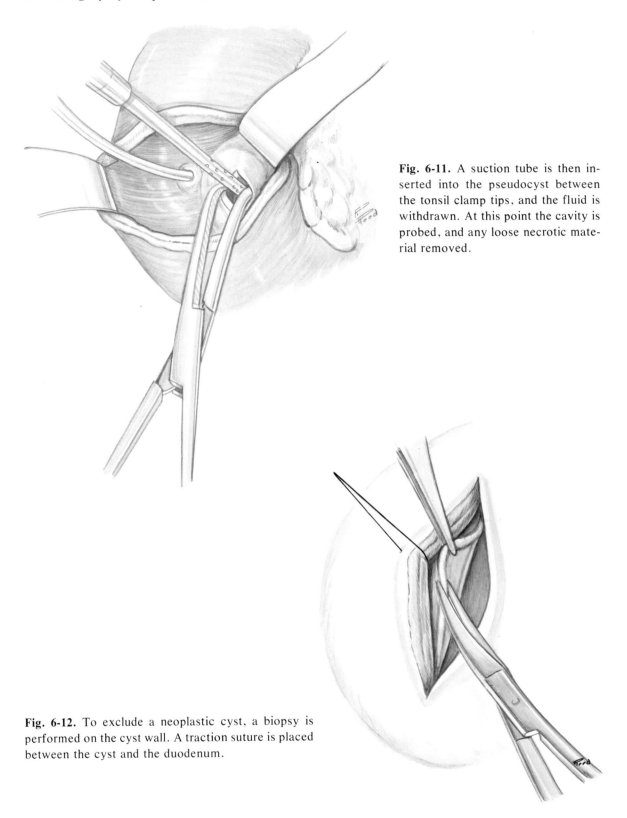

Fig. 6-11. A suction tube is then inserted into the pseudocyst between the tonsil clamp tips, and the fluid is withdrawn. At this point the cavity is probed, and any loose necrotic material removed.

Fig. 6-12. To exclude a neoplastic cyst, a biopsy is performed on the cyst wall. A traction suture is placed between the cyst and the duodenum.

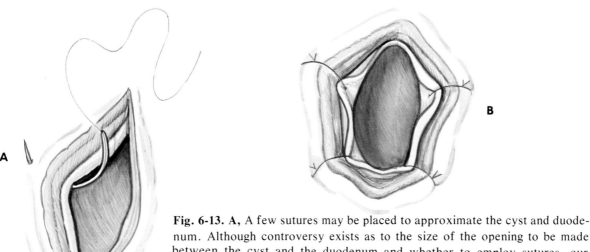

Fig. 6-13. A, A few sutures may be placed to approximate the cyst and duodenum. Although controversy exists as to the size of the opening to be made between the cyst and the duodenum and whether to employ sutures, our impression is that pseudocysts drain by hydrostatic pressure, and when the cyst is empty the opening closes. **B,** The length of opening is 1 to 6 cm. A small incision (2 to 3 cm) has been satisfactory, and this is our preference.

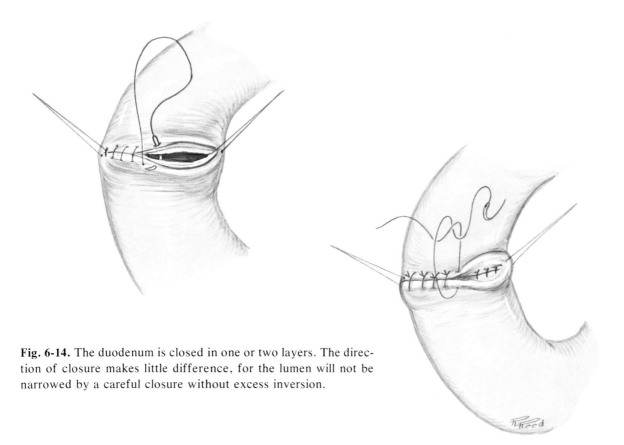

Fig. 6-14. The duodenum is closed in one or two layers. The direction of closure makes little difference, for the lumen will not be narrowed by a careful closure without excess inversion.

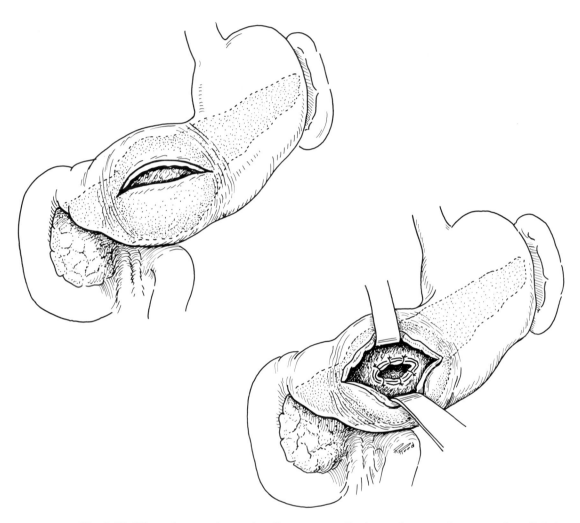

Fig. 6-15. When the pseudocyst is adherent to or displaces the posterior stomach wall, it is drained into the stomach. A longitudinal incision is made in the gastric wall, parallel to the pathway of electrical conduction, and the same steps are followed as in draining the pseudocyst into the duodenum.

Fig. 6-16. In some instances the pseudocyst does not adhere to or approximate the stomach or duodenum. In these instances a loop of jejunum is used. The jejunum is sutured to the cyst side to side.

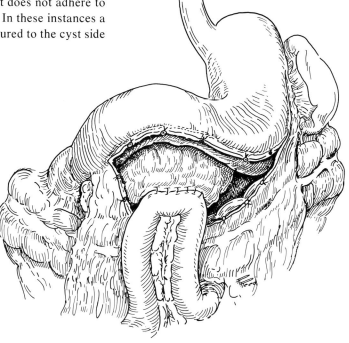

Fig. 6-17. A Roux-en-Y jejunal limb may be used; but this will not be necessary in most instances, since the cyst collapses and probably stops draining in 1 or 2 weeks. We use this method (for technical reasons) when a jejunal loop will not reach the cyst. A jejunojejunostomy is placed beneath the opening to complete the Roux-en-Y anastomosis.

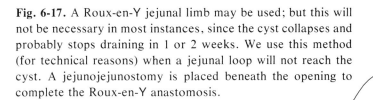

Acute pseudocysts

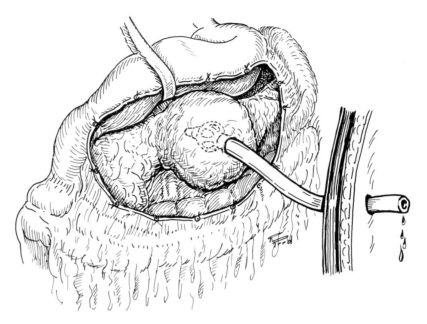

Fig. 6-18. When sepsis and infection mandate early operation and the wall of the pseudo-cyst is friable, external drainage should be done. A catheter is placed in the cavity and brought out through a separate skin opening. About 25% of patients develop a pancreatic fistula. Therefore external drainage will be definitive in 75% of cases. The catheters are left in place until all drainage ceases. A Gastrografin injection is done to estimate the size of the cavity. When the cavity has been closed, the catheters may be removed.

Pseudocyst with biliary obstruction

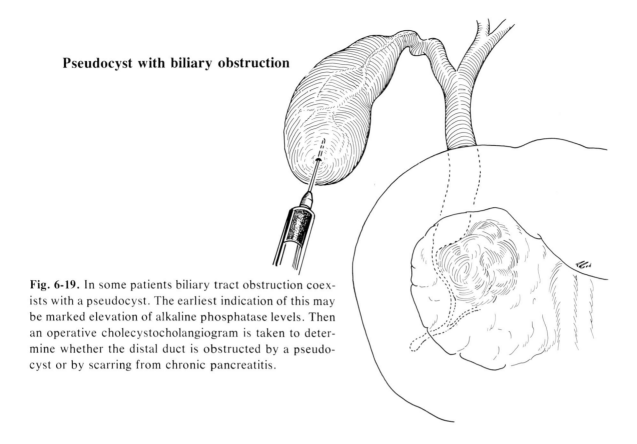

Fig. 6-19. In some patients biliary tract obstruction coexists with a pseudocyst. The earliest indication of this may be marked elevation of alkaline phosphatase levels. Then an operative cholecystocholangiogram is taken to determine whether the distal duct is obstructed by a pseudocyst or by scarring from chronic pancreatitis.

Fig. 6-20. It is important to differentiate between ductal obstruction caused by a pseudocyst and that caused by scarring. In the former instance, drainage of the pseudocyst will relieve the obstruction. If scarring is the cause of the obstruction, a cholecystoenterostomy (in this case a cholecystoduodenostomy) will be necessary.

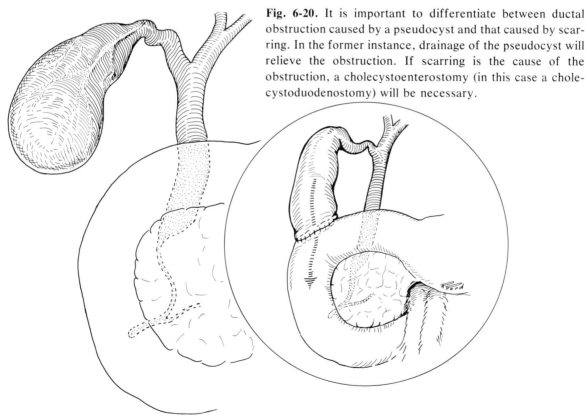

Personal observations

EDWARD L. BRADLEY, III

Since I am in agreement with most of the material contained in this excellent summary, my remarks will emphasize certain features of pseudocysts which we have found to be of particular clinical importance.

Pseudocysts occur much more frequently than previously thought. Sonographic configurations of pseudocyst were found in more than half of ninety-nine patients with severe acute pancreatitis. Although these patients were highly selected with regard to the degree of pancreatitis, peripancreatic collections of fluid appear to be common in such conditions. In the past, patients with nonpalpable pseudocysts have also been underdiagnosed. The newer noninvasive techniques of ultrasonography and computed tomography (CT) have shown increasing numbers of smaller pseudocysts. When these observations are combined with documentation of spontaneous resolution of pseudocysts, the incidence and natural history of pseudocysts may be underreported and inaccurate.

There has also been a great deal of controversy regarding the indications for surgery and the timing of operative intervention in patients with pseudocysts. By means of specific timing criteria, ninety-three patients with a pseudocyst confirmed by ultrasonography were separated into "acute" or "chronic" groups. Of the fifty-two patients classified as acute, progression of the underlying disease or diagnostic uncertainty led to laparotomy in eleven. The remaining forty-one patients were followed by serial sonographic and physical examinations. In ten of these (24%) the pseudocyst underwent spontaneous resolution, whereas in only five (11%) did complications develop which were related to the presence of the pseudocyst (abscess [3], rupture [1], obstructive jaundice [1]). Thirty-one of the patients with a chronic pseudocyst were managed nonoperatively. By contrast, only one (3%) of the chronic pseudocysts underwent spontaneous resolution whereas fifteen (53%) developed complications (rupture [10], abscess [4], obstructive jaundice [1]). Complications in chronic pseudocysts led directly to death in seven cases and occurred an average 13.5 weeks after presumed pseudocyst formation. These observations suggested to us that persistent observation of a pseudocyst in expectation of spontaneous resolution invites unacceptable morbidity and mortality. Since sufficient thickness of the fibrous capsule to permit internal drainage is usually present after 3 to 5 weeks of maturation, laparotomy should be undertaken 5 to 10 weeks after presumed formation, if spontaneous resolution has not taken place before this time.

I too obtain a biopsy of the wall of the pseudocyst since we have encountered four patients with cystic malignancies (cystadenocarcinomas, cystic lymphoma, cystic leiomyosarcoma) that were initially mistaken for pseudocysts.

Although operative cystography may indicate which pseudocyst remains in contact with the pancreatic duct system, I find this procedure to be most useful when multiple cysts are suspected. In these instances I excise a portion of the common wall between the pseudocysts, creating in effect a single chamber. The pseudocyst is then drained into an appropriate segment of intestine (cystojejunostomy or cystogastrostomy). Results with this cloacal technique have been quite satisfactory.

Regarding what type of internal drainage should be done, I agree that cystogastrostomy should be used when the pseudocyst is adherent to the stomach. In this condition I prefer anterior gastrostomy followed by a 2-inch axial incision through the common posterior wall. A running peristomal suture is necessary only if there is bleeding from the stoma. Cystojejunostomy gives equally satisfactory results, but it is a more extensive procedure. We reserve cystojejunostomy for cases in which there is a failure of adherence of the stomach to the pseudocyst or when more dependent drainage may be required for large pseudocysts.

Although cystenteric anastomoses may stay open as long as pancreatic juice drains, I prefer a Roux-en-Y cystojejunostomy to an in-continuity cystojejunostomy. Theoretically, if a cystenteric anastomotic leak occurs, an intestinal fistula will not result if the bowel has been defunctionalized. Our experience with cystoduodenostomy has been voluntarily limited by less favorable results. Like the authors, we reserve this technique for pseudocysts in the head of the pancreas presenting primarily in a posterior direction.

The differentiation between pseudocyst and pancreatitis in obstruction of the common bile duct (Figs. 6-19 and 6-20) is vitally important and has been covered. If abdominal pain is a significant feature of the patient's history and pancreatitis has obstructed the duct, a Whipple procedure may offer the best opportunity for relief. In the absence of abdominal pain, we prefer a choledochoduodenostomy.

REFERENCES

1. Balfour, J. F.: Pancreatic pseudocysts: complications and their relation to the timing of treatment, Surg. Clin. North Am. **50:**395, 1970.
2. Becker, W. F., Pratt, H. S., and Ganji, H.: Pseudocysts of the pancreas, Surg. Gynecol. Obstet. **127:**744, 1968.
3. Bolivar, J. C., and Lempke, R. E.: Pancreatic pseudocyst of the spleen, Ann. Surg. **179:**73, 1974.
4. Bradley, E. L., III, and Clements, J. L., Jr.: Implications of diagnostic ultrasound in the surgical management of pancreatic pseudocysts, Am. J. Surg. **127:**163, 1974.
5. Bradley, E. L., III, and Clements, J. L., Jr.: Spontaneous resolution of pancreatic pseudocysts; implications for timing of operative intervention, Am. J. Surg. **129:**23, 1975.
6. Bradley, E. L., III, Gonzalez, A. C., and Clements, J. L., Jr.: Acute pancreatic pseudocysts, Ann. Surg. **184:**734, 1976.
7. Brewer, W. A., and Shumway, O. L.: Transgastric catheter drainage of pancreatic pseudocysts, Arch. Surg. **78:**79, 1959.
8. Bucknam, C. A.: Arterial hemorrhage in pseudocyst of pancreas, Arch. Surg. **92:**405, 1966.
9. Cerilli, J., and Faris, T. D.: Pancreatic pseudocysts: delayed versus immediate treatment, Surgery **61:**541, 1967.
10. Christensen, N. M., Demling, R., and Mathewson, C., Jr.: Unusual manifestations of pancreatic pseudocysts and their surgical management, Am. J. Surg. **130:**199, 1975.
11. Clauss, R. H., and Wilson, D. W.: Pancreatic pseudocyst of the mediastinum, J. Thorac. Surg. **35:**795, 1951.
12. Cogbill, C. L.: Hemorrhage in pancreatic pseudocysts. Review of literature and report of 2 cases, Ann. Surg. **167:**112, 1967.
13. Cordero, O. C., Khademi, M., Lazaro, E., and Swaminathan, A. P.: Intracystic haemorrhage: a complication of pseudocyst of the pancreas, Br. J. Radiol. **48:**602, 1975.
14. Dardik, I., and Dardik, H.: Patterns of hemorrhage into pancreatic pseudocysts, Am. J. Surg. **115:**774, 1968.
15. Edlin, P.: Mediastinal pseudocyst of the pancreas, Gastroenterology **17:**96, 1951.
16. Folk, F. A., and Freeark, R. J.: Reoperation for pancreatic pseudocysts, Arch. Surg. **100:**430, 1970.
17. Fry, C., Childs, C. G., and Fry, W.: Pancreatectomy for chronic pancreatitis, Ann. Surg. **184:**403, 1976.
18. Goldberg B. B., Lehman, J. S.: Some observations on the practical uses of mode ultrasound, Am. J. Roentgenol. Radium Ther. Nucl. Med. **107:**198, 1969.
19. Gonzalez, L. L., Jaffe, M. S., Wiot, J. F., and Altemeier, W. A.: Pancreatic pseudocyst: a cause of obstructive jaundice, Ann. Surg. **161:**569, 1965.
20. Greenstein, A., DeMaio, E. F., and Nabseth, D. C.: Acute hemorrhage associated with pancreatic pseudocysts, Surgery **69:**56, 1971.
21. Hanna, W. A.: Rupture of pancreatic cysts: report of a case and review of the literature, Br. J. Surg. **47:**495, 1960.
22. Hillson, R. F., and Taube, R. R.: Surgical management of pancreatic pseudocysts. Am. Surg. **41:**492, 1975.
23. Jedlicka, R.: Rozhledy v Chir. a Gynaekol. I. Hft. 3, 1921. Reviewed by Mühlstein, G.: Eine neue Operationsmethode der Pankreacysten (Pancreato-gastrostomie), Zentralbl. Chir. **50:**132, 1923.

24. Lucke, A., and Klebs, E.: Beitrag zur Ovanotome und zur Kenntnis der abdominal Geschwulste, Virchows Arch. Pathol. Anat. **41:**1, 1867.
25. Lutwick, L. I.: Pancreatic abscess with Haemophilus influenzae and Eikenella corrodens, J.A.M.A. **236:**2091, 1976.
26. Parshall, W. A., and ReMine, W. H.: Internal drainage of pseudocysts of the pancreas, Arch. Surg. **91:**480, 1965.
27. Polk, H. C., Jr., Zeppa, R., and Warren, W. D.: Surgical significance of differentiation between acute and chronic pancreatic collections, Ann. Surg. **169:**444, 1969.
28. Reynes, C. J., and Love, L.: Mediastinal pseudocyst, Radiology **92:**115, 1968.
29. Rosenberg, I. K., Kahn, J. A., and Walt, A. J.: Surgical experience with pancreatic pseudocysts, Am. J. Surg. **117:**11, 1969.
30. Shafer, R. B., and Silvis, S. E.: Pancreatic pseudo-pseudocysts, Am. J. Surg. **127:**320, 1974.
31. Sidel, V. W., Wilson, R. E., and Shipp, J. C.: Pseudocyst formation in chronic pancreatitis: a cause of obstructive jaundice, Arch. Surg. **77:**933, 1958
32. Sybers, H. D., Shelp, W. D., and Morrissey, J. F.: Pseudocyst of the pancreas with fistulous extension into the neck, N. Engl. J. Med. **278:**1058, 1968.
33. Vajcner, A., and Nicoloff, D. M.: Pseudocysts of the pancreas: value of urine and serum amylase levels, Surgery **66:**842, 1969.
34. van Heerden, J. A., and ReMine, W. H.: Pseudocysts of the pancreas. Review of 71 cases, Arch. Surg. **110:**500, 1975.
35. Van Nostrand, W. R., Renert, W. A., and Hileman, W. T.: Milk-of-calcium of the pancreas, Radiology **110:**323, 1974.
36. Warren, K. W., Athanassiades, S., Frederick, P., and Kune, G. A.: Surgical treatment of pancreatic cysts: review of 183 cases, Ann. Surg. **163:**886, 1966.
37. Warren, W. D., Marsh, W. H., and Muller, W. H., Jr.: Experimental production of pseudocysts of the pancreas with preliminary observations of internal drainage, Surg. Gynecol. Obstet. **105:**385, 1957.
38. Weinstein, B. R., Korn, R. J., and Zimmerman, H. J.: Obstructive jaundice as a complication of pancreatitis, Ann. Intern. Med. **58:**245, 1963.

CHAPTER 7

Chronic pancreatitis: an overview

ROBERT E. HERMANN

The Marseilles Symposium on Pancreatitis in 1963 proposed that
patients with pancreatitis be classified into four groups[10]: (1) acute pancreatitis, when the attack is the initial episode, (2) recurrent acute pancreatitis, when the attack is a secondary or subsequent episode, (3) recurrent
chronic pancreatitis, when many episodes occur over a period of years and
evidence of fibrosis or calcification is found at operation, and (4) chronic
pancreatitis, when the episodes are virtually continuous or when weight
loss, steatorrhea, diabetes mellitus, or narcotic addiction is a problem.

Pancreatitis is a recurring and progressive disease in 53% to 90% of
patients depending on the cause of the disease and the treatment available.[2,4,8] It is not surprising that recurrent episodes of acute pancreatitis
cause progressive fibrosis and inflammatory changes in the pancreas
leading to chronic pancreatitis. The percentage of patients with acute
pancreatitis who have recurring episodes relates more closely to the
etiology of the disease than to any other factor. If cholecystitis is the cause
of a single episode of acute pancreatitis, cholecystectomy can correct the
condition and recurrent episodes of pancreatitis are unlikely to occur. If
the cause of the pancreatitis is alcoholism, then recurring episodes of
pancreatic inflammation will be most likely related to the drinking habits
of the patient.

Alcoholism is the leading cause of *chronic* pancreatitis. Other less
frequent causes are biliary tract disease, peptic ulcers, idiopathic (no
known cause), hyperlipemia, and congenital abnormalities of the pancreatic duct system.[5] Congenital abnormalities of the pancreatic duct system
are one cause that has only recently been recognized with the advent of
pancreatography. Some patients with idiopathic pancreatitis have congeni-

116

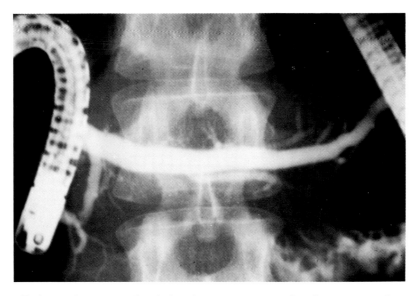

Fig. 7-1. Endoscopic retrograde cholangiopancreatogram showing presumed congenital stenosis of the pancreatic duct (partially obscured by the radiopaque endoscope) in a 22-year-old man, who had had several episodes of recurrent acute pancreatitis.

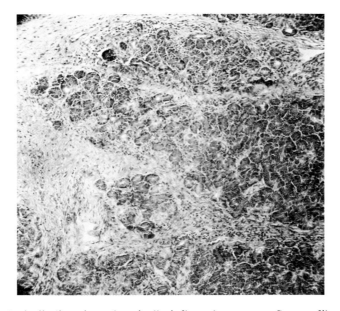

Fig. 7-2. Histologic findings in a chronically inflamed pancreas. Severe fibrosis gradually replaces the normal glandular architecture.

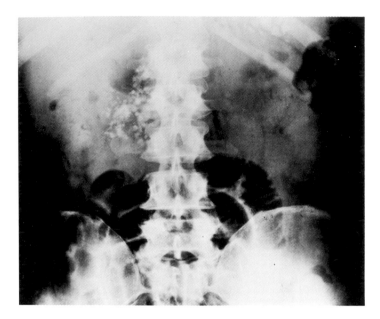

Fig. 7-3. Plain roentgenogram of the abdomen showing multiple calcifications in the region of the pancreas.

tal stenosis of the pancreatic duct system, which may be difficult to recognize since ductal stenosis is both a result and a possible cause of chronic pancreatitis (Fig. 7-1).

The major clinical symptoms associated with chronic pancreatitis and those that impel the patient to seek medical attention are severe pain in the epigastrium radiating into the back, nausea and vomiting, gradual weight loss, steatorrhea, and diabetes mellitus. Pseudocysts of the pancreas can occur in patients with chronic pancreatitis as well as in patients with acute pancreatitis.[6]

Histologic findings in patients with chronic pancreatitis include fibrosis and thickening of the gland, dilatation of the pancreatic duct system with multiple areas of stenosis and stricture formation, calcium carbonate deposits within the gland as a result of the chronic inflammation, atrophy of the acinar cells, and eventual atrophy or destruction of the islet cells (Fig. 7-2). Most of the calcifications in chronic pancreatitis leading to further irritation and blockage of the ducts are found in the pancreatic duct system (Fig. 7-3). Often flecks of calcium can be expressed from secondary and tertiary ducts at operative exploration of the pancreas. In the majority of patients, recurring episodes of pancreatitis leading to chronic pancreatitis are believed to be related to partial or intermittent episodes of pancreatic duct obstruction.[1,3,7,9] Because chronic pancreatitis itself causes pancreatic duct stenosis, it becomes a self-perpetuating disease.

OPERATIVE MANAGEMENT

A variety of surgical procedures has been used to treat recurrent chronic and chronic pancreatitis. These procedures include direct surgery on the pancreas as well as surgical procedures on other organs thought to be causally related to the recurring disease.[6]

When uncorrected biliary disease can be identified and is thought to be the cause of recurrent or chronic pancreatitis, operations on the biliary system are often of great value. These include cholecystectomy, common bile duct exploration with removal of stones, sphincteroplasty for stenosis of the sphincter of Oddi, and biliary enteric bypass when distal biliary obstruction cannot be corrected by sphincteroplasty. When peptic ulcer is thought to be a cause of pancreatitis, an operation for duodenal ulcer has been used effectively. When hyperparathyroidism has been identified as a cause of recurrent pancreatitis, parathyroidectomy is performed. Gastrojejunostomy alone or combined with vagotomy has been used for duodenal stenosis or obstruction secondary to recurrent or chronic pancreatitis.

Operations on the pancreas have included transduodenal sphincteroplasty with exploration of the pancreatic duct and curettage and removal of calcifications, longitudinal pancreaticojejunostomy, distal pancreatectomy with or without pancreaticojejunostomy, pancreaticoduodenal resection, and radical subtotal pancreatectomy preserving only a margin of pancreas along the common bile duct and duodenum. In some patients who have a pseudocyst of the pancreas associated with chronic pancreatitis, a drainage of the pseudocyst by means of cystogastrostomy, cystojejunostomy, or cystoduodenostomy is first done. Finally, when continuing pain radiating into the back seems out of proportion to the severity or extent of the disease in the pancreas or the surgeon is reluctant to remove the pancreas for whatever reason, and when pancreatic duct drainage procedures have failed, splanchnic resection can be performed to divide the splanchnic nerves and provide relief of pain (Chapter 8).

The timing of operations for pancreatitis is important. Since pancreatitis is a disease with intermittent acute episodes of inflammation which subside on medical therapy, we believe that with rare exception operations on the acutely inflamed gland are contraindicated. Acute flareups occur in patients with chronic pancreatitis as well as in patients with acute recurrent pancreatitis. Therefore, when any patient with an acute episode is admitted to the hospital it is important initially to treat the patient medically and abort the inflammatory process. Whenever possible, we try to plan elective operations on patients with chronic pancreatitis during a period when the disease is relatively quiescent.

The key to the operative management of chronic pancreatitis is individualization: assess the likely etiologic factors and correct them if possible. This means that the patient's history, the findings on physical examination, the results of laboratory studies, and the findings of routine and special roentgenographic studies must all be given careful attention. At the time of operation, careful inspection and evaluation of the biliary system, stomach, duodenum, and other intra-abdominal organs must be carried out. Operative cholangiography is frequently desirable, especially if preoperative cholangiographic studies are not clearly normal.

Data comparing operations for pancreatitis are uncontrolled and difficult to assess. Follow-up information and selection of patients and operations are based on the individual surgeon's preference. We believe that the operative pancreatogram is of great value in helping decide what operative procedure should be performed on the pancreas and is probably the best guide to the treatment of chronic pancreatitis. If pancreatic duct obstruction is identified by operative pancreatography, the obstruction should be relieved. If the duct is dilated but the gland is too diseased to be treated by decompression of the duct alone, then the surgeon may, in addition, choose to resect a portion of the gland (Fig. 7-4). If the operative pancreatogram shows no evidence of duct dilatation but fibrosis and calcification of the gland predominate, then pancreatic resection alone should be employed. Whether the head of the pancreas should be resected by pancreaticoduodenectomy or whether the distal pancreas should be resected, and how much, depends mainly on the severity of the disease diagnosed preoperatively, the findings encountered at surgery, and the findings of operative pancreatography.

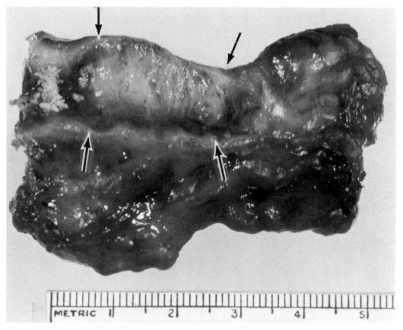

Fig. 7-4. A pancreatic resection has been done. Note the large dilated duct (arrows) containing calculi.

Surgical techniques

The techniques of direct surgical procedures on the pancreas which we have utilized at the Cleveland Clinic during the past fifteen years are described.

Transduodenal sphincteroplasty and exploration of the pancreatic duct
(Figs. 7-5 to 7-14)

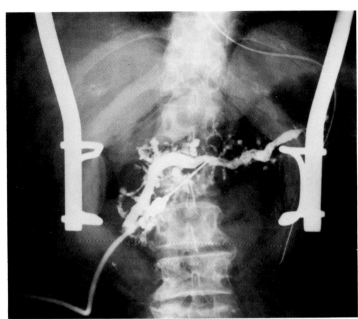

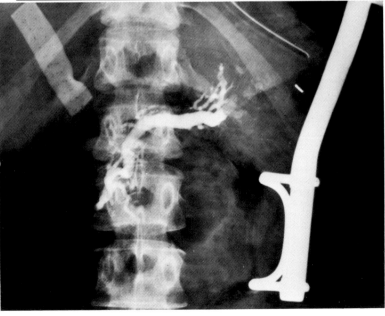

Fig. 7-5. Operative pancreatograms representative of those that show stenosis of the pancreatic duct opening into the duodenum with dilatation of the duct. This roentgenographic evidence of fibrosis of the pancreatic duct opening is an indication for sphincteroplasty.

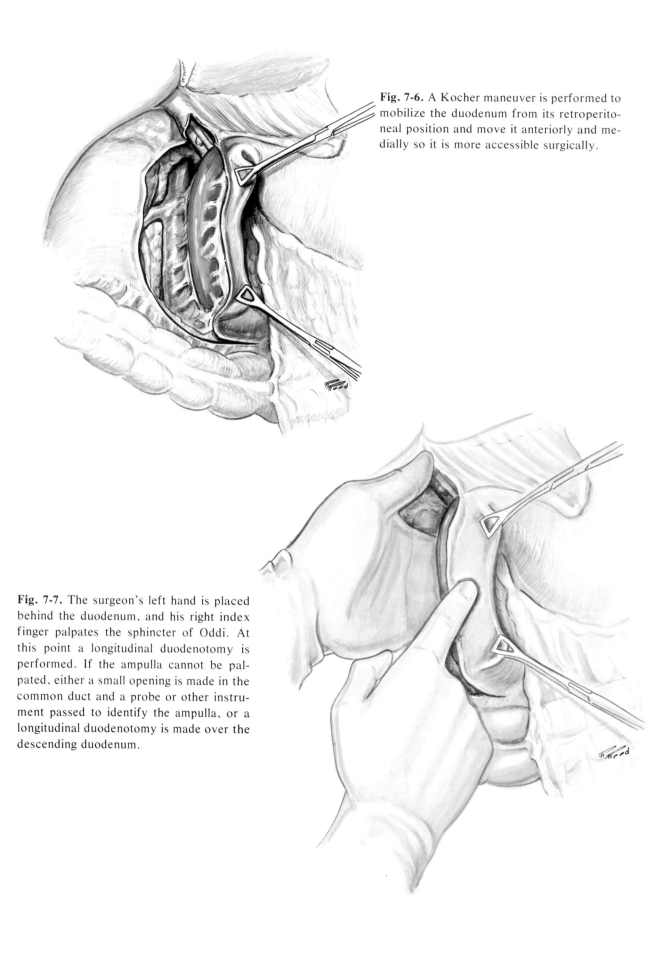

Fig. 7-6. A Kocher maneuver is performed to mobilize the duodenum from its retroperitoneal position and move it anteriorly and medially so it is more accessible surgically.

Fig. 7-7. The surgeon's left hand is placed behind the duodenum, and his right index finger palpates the sphincter of Oddi. At this point a longitudinal duodenotomy is performed. If the ampulla cannot be palpated, either a small opening is made in the common duct and a probe or other instrument passed to identify the ampulla, or a longitudinal duodenotomy is made over the descending duodenum.

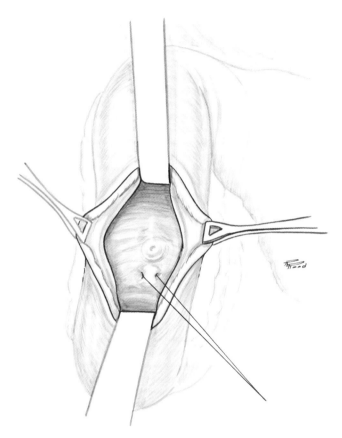

Fig. 7-8. A longitudinal duodenotomy has been performed and small right-angled retractors are placed in the duodenum to expose the medial wall and the papilla of Vater. A traction suture of 3-0 silk is placed in the medial wall of the duodenum below the papilla to bring the duodenal wall anteriorly and aid in exposure.

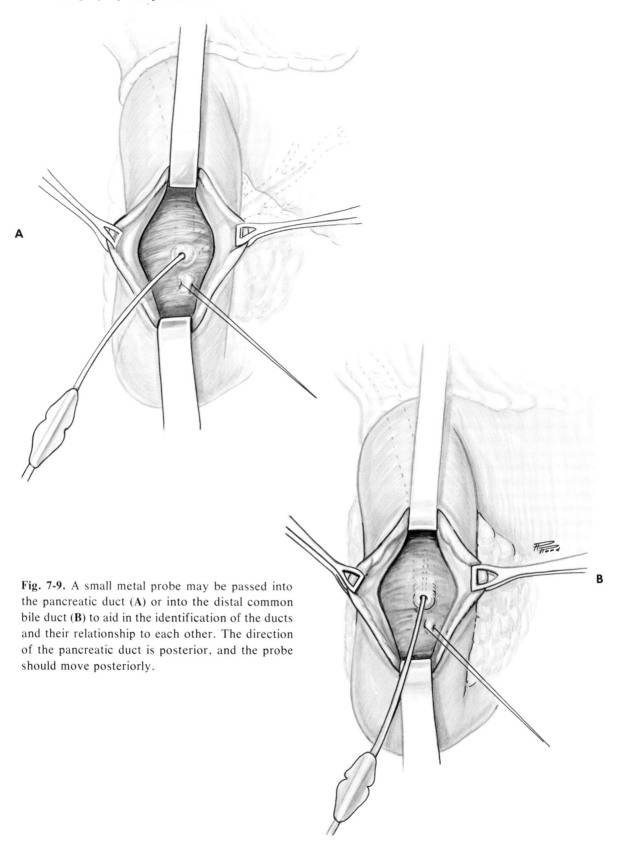

Fig. 7-9. A small metal probe may be passed into the pancreatic duct (**A**) or into the distal common bile duct (**B**) to aid in the identification of the ducts and their relationship to each other. The direction of the pancreatic duct is posterior, and the probe should move posteriorly.

Fig. 7-10. Using an angled vascular scissors, the surgeon cuts the sphincter of Oddi at 11 o'clock for a distance of 1.5 to 2.5 cm. The location of this incision into the ampulla of Vater is important to avoid injury to the pancreatic duct opening.

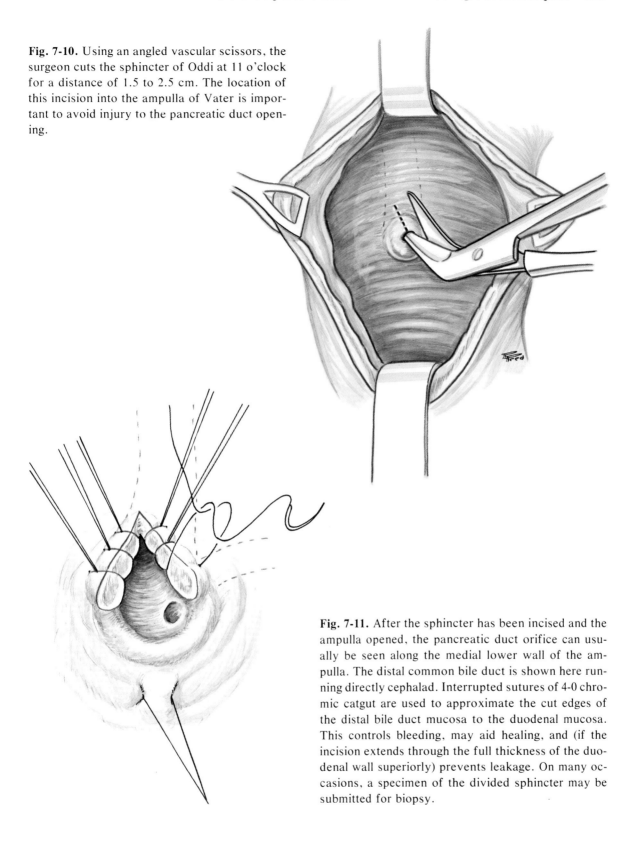

Fig. 7-11. After the sphincter has been incised and the ampulla opened, the pancreatic duct orifice can usually be seen along the medial lower wall of the ampulla. The distal common bile duct is shown here running directly cephalad. Interrupted sutures of 4-0 chromic catgut are used to approximate the cut edges of the distal bile duct mucosa to the duodenal mucosa. This controls bleeding, may aid healing, and (if the incision extends through the full thickness of the duodenal wall superiorly) prevents leakage. On many occasions, a specimen of the divided sphincter may be submitted for biopsy.

Fig. 7-12. Close-up magnified view of the completed choledochal sphincteroplasty. The surgeon now cuts the septum between the common bile duct and pancreatic duct, incising the stenotic pancreatic duct opening. Again a triangular segment may be submitted for biopsy. This enlarges the pancreatic duct opening.

If the pancreatic duct orifice is difficult to identify, careful probing with lacrimal duct probes may help locate it. A small amount of secretin can be given intravenously to stimulate pancreatic secretion. The surgeon then looks for droplets of clear watery pancreatic juice in the ampulla or the surrounding duodenal mucosa. With increasing experience in locating the pancreatic duct opening, he may find this rarely necessary.

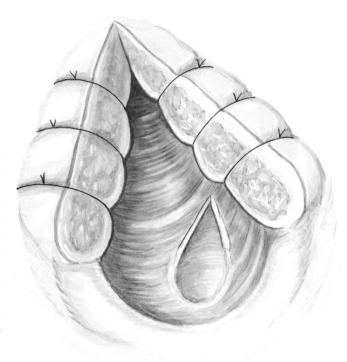

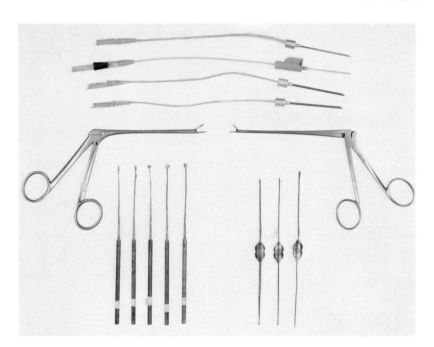

Fig. 7-13. Some of the instruments I use for exploring the pancreatic duct. Included are four catheters with needles (to be removed before the duct is catheterized), two long rongeurs for crushing and extracting stones, fine wire loops (five graded sizes), and three lacrimal duct probes.

After sphincteroplasty the pancreatic duct opening is evident and the duct is progressively dilated with tonsil clamps or Kelly clamps. Probes, loops, and rongeurs are then passed and all accessible stones and debris are removed from the duct. The duct is then irrigated with saline solution introduced through a plastic catheter.

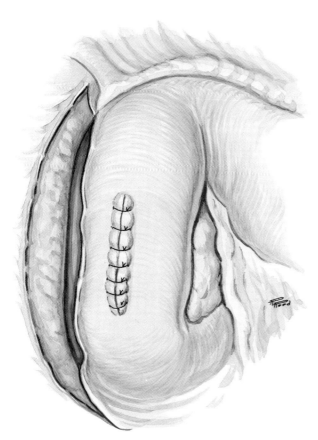

Fig. 7-14. The surgeon closes the duodenotomy in two layers using a continuous inverting suture of 3-0 chromic catgut for the mucosa and submucosa and interrupted 3-0 silk sutures for the seromuscular outer layer.

The duodenotomy and pancreas are not drained.

The gallbladder is removed as a complementary procedure in most patients who have had a sphincteroplasty, even if there is no evidence of biliary disease, to exclude small stones in the gallbladder which may be missed by cholangiography or palpation at surgery.

A T-tube is placed in the common bile duct for postoperative drainage only if the duct has been explored through a separate choledochotomy incision.

Longitudinal pancreaticojejunostomy (modified Puestow procedure) (Figs. 7-15 to 7-24)

Fig. 7-15. The surgeon approaches the pancreas and usually exposes it throughout its length by dividing the gastrocolic omentum, preserving the gastroepiploic vessels along the greater curvature of the stomach. He then enters the lesser peritoneal cavity and explores the pancreas. At times downward traction on the stomach and incision of the gastrohepatic omentum will expose the neck and body of the pancreas and provide access to the duct (not shown) in this area.

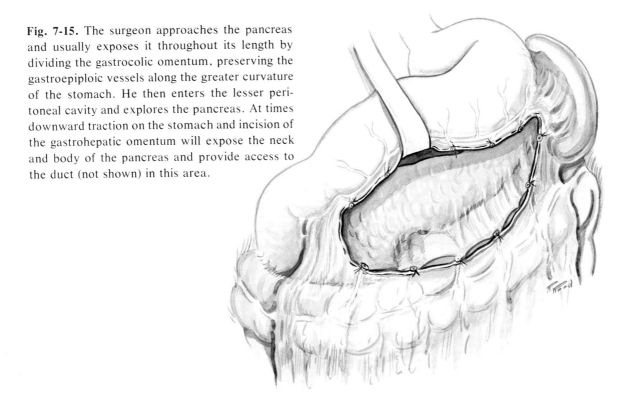

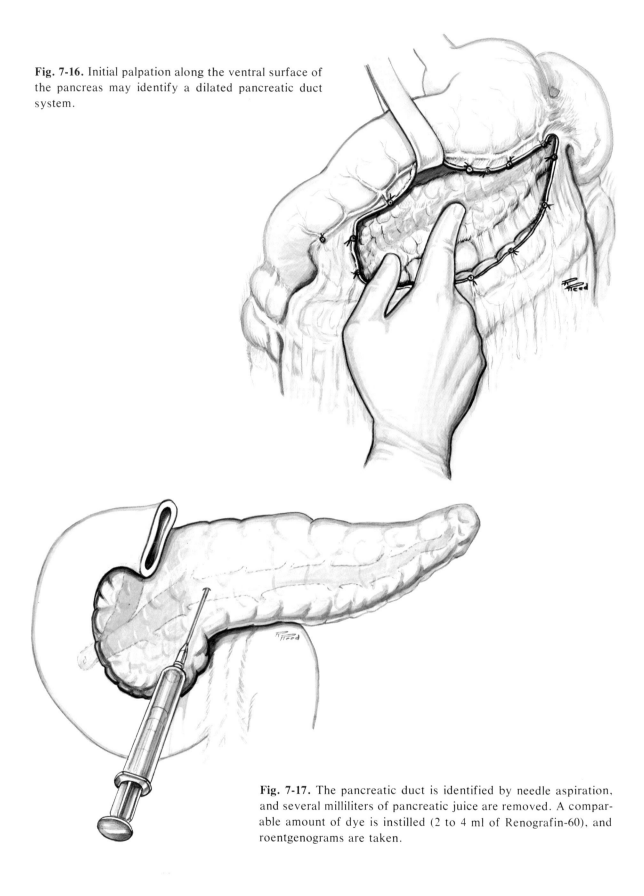

Fig. 7-16. Initial palpation along the ventral surface of the pancreas may identify a dilated pancreatic duct system.

Fig. 7-17. The pancreatic duct is identified by needle aspiration, and several milliliters of pancreatic juice are removed. A comparable amount of dye is instilled (2 to 4 ml of Renografin-60), and roentgenograms are taken.

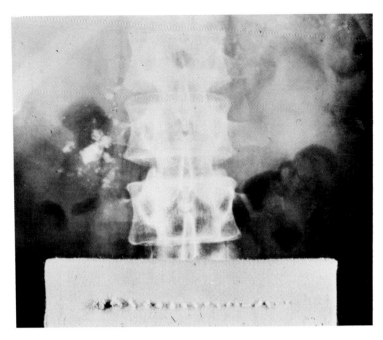

Fig. 7-18. Pancreatic calculi removed at operation demonstrated on a preoperative plain abdominal roentgenogram.

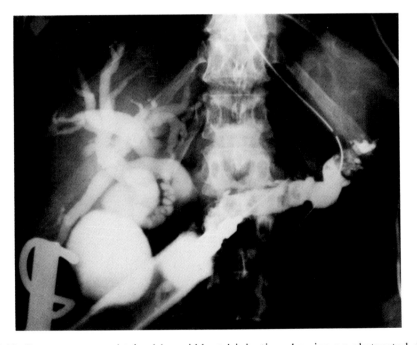

Fig. 7-19. Pancreatogram obtained by midductal injection showing an obstructed dilated pancreatic duct. A longitudinal pancreaticojejunostomy was deemed the best method of decompression. A separately obtained cholecystocholangiogram showed dilatation of the biliary ductal systems.

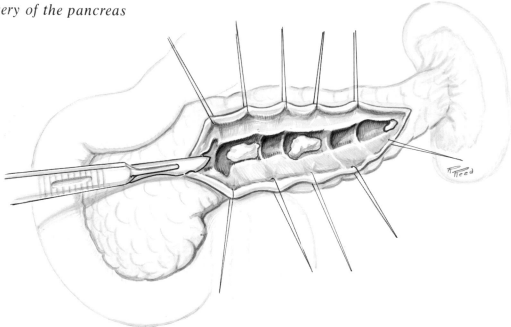

Fig. 7-20. The pancreas is incised longitudinally, over the dilated duct, and the duct is opened. A segment of pancreatic tissue along the ventral surface is excised for biopsy study. Traction sutures of 3-0 silk or synthetic absorbable suture material are used along the opened duct. Stones are seen in the pancreatic ducts. The duct is opened widely throughout its length, and all stones or calculi are removed.

Fig. 7-21. A Roux-en-Y jejunal segment is then fashioned with an 8-to-12-inch proximal segment and a defunctionalized distal segment of approximately 18 inches.

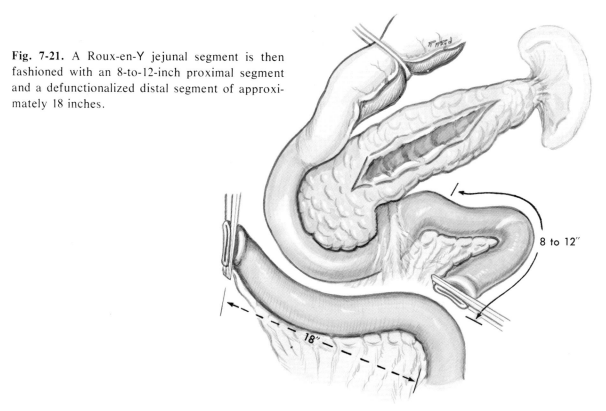

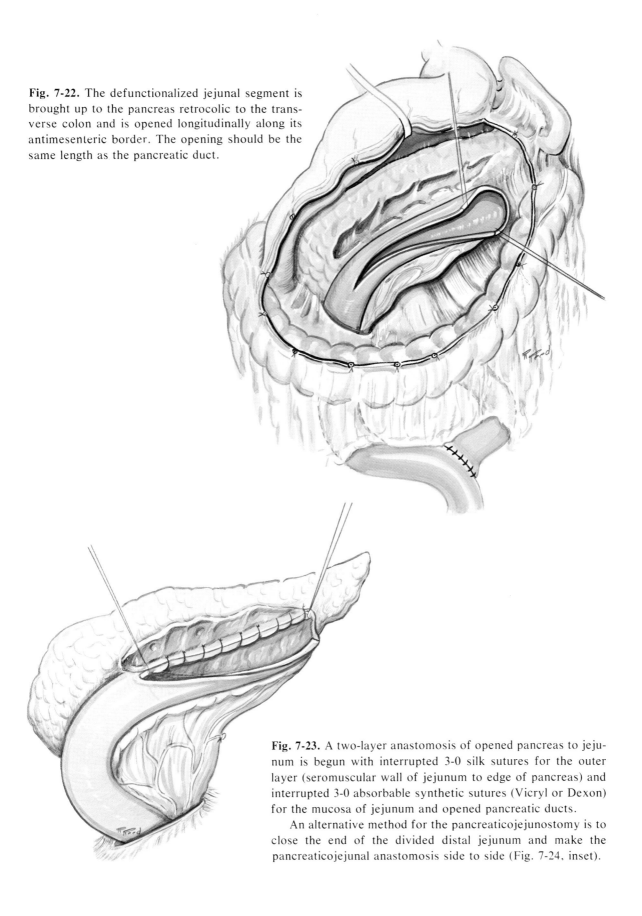

Fig. 7-22. The defunctionalized jejunal segment is brought up to the pancreas retrocolic to the transverse colon and is opened longitudinally along its antimesenteric border. The opening should be the same length as the pancreatic duct.

Fig. 7-23. A two-layer anastomosis of opened pancreas to jejunum is begun with interrupted 3-0 silk sutures for the outer layer (seromuscular wall of jejunum to edge of pancreas) and interrupted 3-0 absorbable synthetic sutures (Vicryl or Dexon) for the mucosa of jejunum and opened pancreatic ducts.

An alternative method for the pancreaticojejunostomy is to close the end of the divided distal jejunum and make the pancreaticojejunal anastomosis side to side (Fig. 7-24, inset).

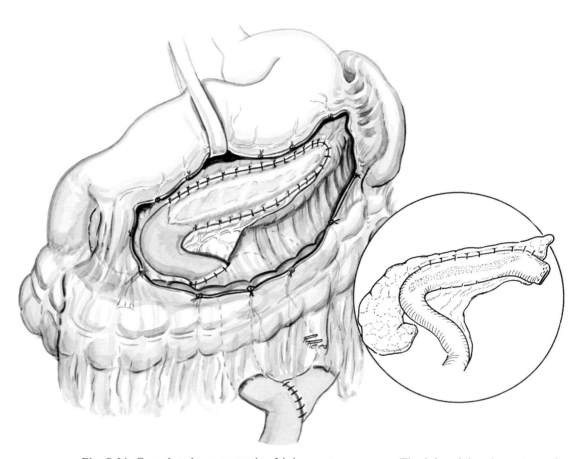

Fig. 7-24. Completed anastomosis of jejunum to pancreas. The jejunojejunal anastomosis is then completed in two layers with silk and chromic catgut sutures or an autosuture. The pancreatic anastomosis is drained by a sump suction catheter left in place for about 5 days. Antibiotics are not given to most patients before or during surgery. (Inset shows the end of the jejunum closed and a side-to-side anastomosis.)

Distal pancreatectomy with or without pancreaticojejunostomy (Figs. 7-25 to 7-33)

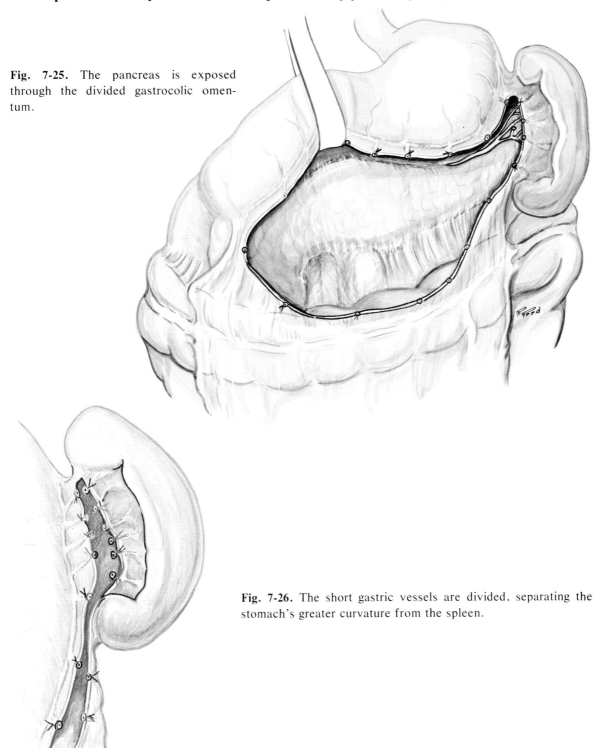

Fig. 7-25. The pancreas is exposed through the divided gastrocolic omentum.

Fig. 7-26. The short gastric vessels are divided, separating the stomach's greater curvature from the spleen.

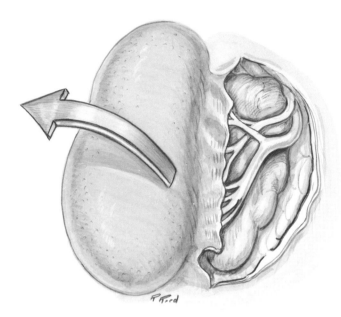

Fig. 7-27. The spleen is mobilized anteriorly, and its posterolateral peritoneal attachments are divided. As it is mobilized anteriorly and medially, the tail of the pancreas is visualized and mobilized anteriorly as well.

The spleen is then resected; and as it is mobilized forward, the splenic artery and vein are ligated from behind the pancreas.

Fig. 7-28. Mobilization of the pancreas up out of its retroperitoneal bed continues by blunt and sharp dissection in the usually avascular plane behind the gland.

The surgeon divides peritoneum above and below the pancreas along the edge of the gland, working from left to right, as he mobilizes the gland.

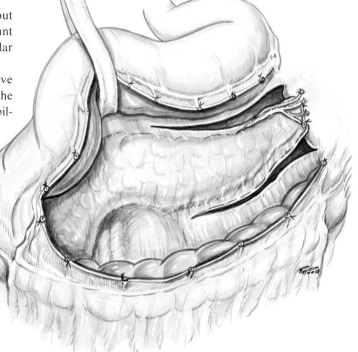

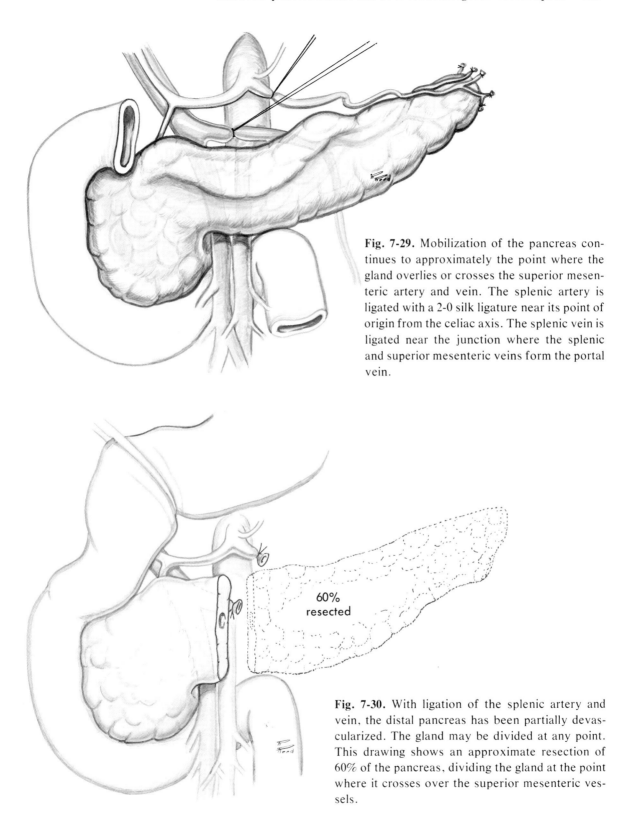

Fig. 7-29. Mobilization of the pancreas continues to approximately the point where the gland overlies or crosses the superior mesenteric artery and vein. The splenic artery is ligated with a 2-0 silk ligature near its point of origin from the celiac axis. The splenic vein is ligated near the junction where the splenic and superior mesenteric veins form the portal vein.

60%
resected

Fig. 7-30. With ligation of the splenic artery and vein, the distal pancreas has been partially devascularized. The gland may be divided at any point. This drawing shows an approximate resection of 60% of the pancreas, dividing the gland at the point where it crosses over the superior mesenteric vessels.

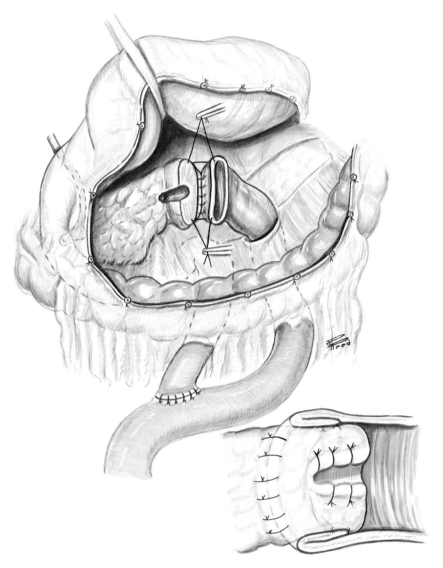

Fig. 7-31. Main features of a distal pancreaticojejunostomy. The distal pancreatic duct is opened, and a two-layer anastomosis made between distal pancreas and a Roux-en-Y jejunal segment. The distal pancreas is stuffed into the end of the jejunum. Silk sutures are used for the outer layer of this anastomosis, absorbable synthetic sutures for the inner mucosal layer. This anastomosis permits retrograde drainage if the proximal pancreatic duct is obstructed. The lower figure is a longitudinal section showing the opened pancreatic duct sutured to adjoining pancreatic tissue.

The distal pancreaticojejunostomy is employed when distal pancreas is diseased and the proximal duct dilated and uniform in diameter.

Fig. 7-32. If a larger portion of the pancreas must be resected because of more extensive disease, retroperitoneal mobilization of the pancreas (from the tail toward the head) is continued. If the pancreas is dissected away from the superior mesenteric vein, great care must be taken to ligate carefully all venous tributaries to that vein.

As the surgeon approaches the common bile duct, he can identify its location by passing a metal probe into the duct to aid in avoiding bile duct injury. The gastroduodenal artery and superior pancreaticoduodenal branches should be protected to preserve the blood supply of the duodenum. These can be identified and will serve as landmarks for the dissection.

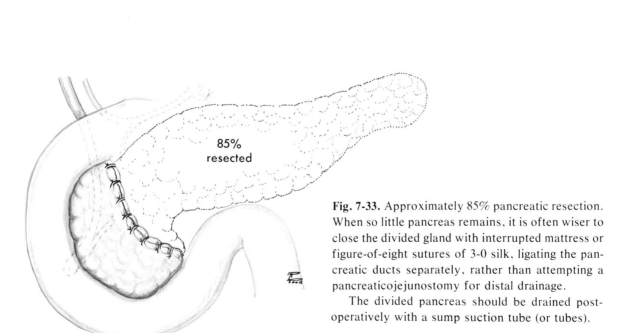

85%
resected

Fig. 7-33. Approximately 85% pancreatic resection. When so little pancreas remains, it is often wiser to close the divided gland with interrupted mattress or figure-of-eight sutures of 3-0 silk, ligating the pancreatic ducts separately, rather than attempting a pancreaticojejunostomy for distal drainage.

The divided pancreas should be drained postoperatively with a sump suction tube (or tubes).

Personal observations

STANLEY O. HOERR

In the past forty years a wide variety of operative procedures has been offered to the profession by surgeons dealing with so-called "chronic pancreatitis." These have varied from a simple biliary bypass procedure (very effective if the only symptom is obstructive jaundice) to total pancreatectomy (the ultimate solution, now generally abandoned since it substitutes unfailingly a "brittle diabetes" and enzymatic insufficiency for whatever symptoms the disease was producing).

Recognizing that in many patients pain is the principal disabling complaint, some authors have recommended splanchnicectomy. Although this may still be useful in particular circumstances today, unfortunately in most patients if the pancreatic inflammation does not burn itself out there seems to be an escape mechanism resulting in the recurrence of pain after an interval of months to years.

One of the problems in improving our understanding of pancreatic inflammation has been the failure to distinguish clinical forms of the disease. At one end of the spectrum is the single acute attack of pancreatitis; at the other end, the incapacitating continuous pain suffered by patients with advanced chronic pancreatitis. As Dr. Hermann notes, the classification proposed at the Marseilles Symposium in 1963 has done much to clarify our thinking and our reporting.

A second problem in the past has been a failure to distinguish the different etiologies that may produce the same end result: for example, obstruction of the principal pancreatic duct by stone and fibrosis, which produces both pain and steatorrhea and is correctable by proper decompression of the ductal system, being confused with pancreatic cirrhosis, in which diffuse involvement of the gland does not permit such a simple solution.

It has long been known that chronic pancreatitis is particularly intractable in alcoholics; and yet a morphologically and clinically indistinguishable form of the disease may occur in patients who, so far as can be determined, have never touched a drop of spirits. There is also the puzzling finding of pancreatic calcification on abdominal roentgenograms of patients who have no current symptoms relating to the pancreas and cannot recall ever having had such symptoms in the past!

The surgeon who has a patient with either "recurrent chronic pancreatitis" (i.e., symptom-free intervals between attacks but with fibrosis presumably progressing in the gland) or true "chronic pancreatitis" (pain and other symptoms more or less constant) should first be certain that all conservative (nonsurgical) measures have been exhausted. If operative intervention is deemed warranted, the *least extensive procedure which promises relief* should be considered; if it fails, further surgery can always be done. Pancreatography helps the surgeon decide which operation will be the best.

Chronic pancreatitis producing painless jaundice may be indistinguishable at the operating table from carcinoma of the head of the pancreas; a biliary bypass is all that should be done. If obstruction of the pancreatic duct can be demonstrated by operative pancreatography, some type of decompression must be achieved; this may be accomplished by a sphincteroplasty, but in most cases will require an anastomosis between the pancreatic duct and the small intestine with or without resection of the distal pancreas. Rarely with such pancreatitis will stones in the common bile duct appear to be the initiating pathology; but if so simple a cause can be discovered, choledocholithotomy may be all that should be done. Only rarely should radical subtotal (95%) pancreatectomy be considered as a first procedure.

In summary, surgical intervention for chronic pancreatitis should address itself to the least risky or extensive procedure which gives fair promise of relieving symptoms. Since chronic pancreatitis is only rarely fatal in and of itself, relief of symptoms rather than cure of the disease is a legitimate therapeutic goal.

REFERENCES

1. Bartlett, M. K., and Nardi, G. L.: Treatment of recurrent pancreatitis by transduodenal sphincterotomy and exploration of pancreatic duct, N. Engl. J. Med. **262:**643, 1960.
2. Dreiling, D. A., Janowitz, H. D., and Perrier, C. V.: Pancreatic inflammatory disease; a physiologic approach, New York, 1964, Paul B. Hoeber, Inc.
3. Farrell, J. J., Richmond, K. C., and Morgan, M. M.: Transduodenal pancreatic duct dilatation and curettage in chronic relapsing pancreatitis, Am. J. Surg. **105:**30, 1963.
4. Fitzgerald, O., Fitzgerald, P., and McMullin, J. P.: Chronic pancreatitis; a review, Rev. Surg. **21:**77, 1964.
5. Hermann, R. E.: Basic factors in the pathogenesis of pancreatitis, Cleve. Clin. Q. **30:**1, 1963.
6. Hermann, R. E., Al-Jurf, A. S., and Hoerr, S. O.: Pancreatitis; surgical management, Arch. Surg. **109:**298, 1974.
7. Hermann, R. E., and Davis, J. H.: The role of incomplete pancreatic duct obstruction in the etiology of pancreatitis, Surgery **48:**318, 1960.
8. Howard, J. M., and James, P. M.: Pancreatitis; a survey of its current status, Rev. Surg. **19:**301, 1962.
9. Howard, J. M., and Nedwich, A.: Correlation of the histologic observations and operative findings in patients with chronic pancreatitis, Surg. Gynecol. Obstet. **132:**387, 1971.
10. Sarles, H., and Camatte, R.: Pancréatites aigues; conceptions et therapeutiques recentes, Paris, 1963, Masson & Cie.
11. Stobbe, K. C., ReMine, W. C., and Baggenstoss, A. H.: Pancreatic lithiasis, Surg. Gynecol. Obstet. **131:**1090, 1970.

CHAPTER 8

Thoracic splanchnicectomy and sympathectomy for relief of pancreatic pain

EDWARD S. SADAR
RUSSELL W. HARDY, Jr.

The concept of denervation procedures for the relief of pain of pancreatic disease began with the investigations of the innervation of the pancreas. These early works, experimental and clinical, provided both the substrate for our present palliative surgical procedures and the beginning of controversy regarding the type of procedure best employed.

By the time of Richin's[9] work on the innervation of the pancreas, it was accepted that the nerves which enter the pancreas include sympathetic, parasympathetic, and afferent components, all of which pass through the celiac plexus and reach the gland via the blood vessels supplying it. The afferent pathways of these nerves, their role in the conduction of painful sensation arising in the abdominal viscera, and the results of various ablative procedures were still undefined.

The works by Ray and Neill[8] in 1947 and Bingham and co-workers[1] in 1950 summarized the historical perspective, the anatomic facts, and the clinical experimental studies on which we have based our procedure for the treatment of intractable pancreatic pain. Since 1950 we have been successfully performing bilateral thoracic sympathectomies and splanchnicectomies as the treatment of choice for the intractable pain of pancreatic carcinoma and at times for chronic pancreatitis.[5,10]

In this chapter we explain our rationale for choice of patients, comment on alternative techniques, and illustrate our surgical technique as adapted from that of Peet in 1935.[7]

Whenever a patient has abdominal and/or back pain which might be caused by pancreatic disease, a neurosurgeon participates in the preoperative evaluation. If it is not felt that a laparotomy will result in the relief of pain, for example by removal of an obstruction or resection of a localized disease process, the patient is examined physically and psychologically as a potential candidate for a bilateral thoracic splanchnicectomy-sympathectomy to be done in tandem with a laparotomy.

Psychologic problems are not usually encountered with pancreatic carcinoma but rather with chronic pancreatitis and its associated problems of addiction to alcohol and other pain-relieving medications. If a patient has an appropriate response to repetitive bilateral lidocaine blocks of the paravertebral sympathetic chains and splanchnic nerves at the proposed surgical level (T-11), he is considered a candidate for surgery. Addiction alone has not been a contraindication to surgery, because the problems of addiction would be virtually insurmountable if relief of pain could not be accomplished first. An addict with an inappropriate response to lidocaine blocks or a differential spinal anesthesia (e.g., exaggeration of pain) would not be a surgical candidate. Finally, because we have encountered patients with pancreatic carcinoma whose pain has been relieved surgically but not by prior diagnostic blocks, we have been reluctant to refuse potentially palliative surgery because of a nondiagnostic block in a patient with pancreatic carcinoma, as long as the patient is aware of the decisional dilemma which we face.

There are alternatives to open surgical ablative procedures. A 50% solution of alcohol or a 60% solution of phenol can be used percutaneously[4] or intraoperatively[3] while the celiac ganglion is exposed. Lack of long-term follow-up and inadequate definition of a "good result" have made direct comparison of these reported series with our own results impossible. Appreciating the difficulties of obtaining even temporary adequate preoperative diagnostic blocks, and of surgically isolating the celiac ganglion in the presence of many pancreatic tumors, we have not used these procedures ourselves. For more information, the reader is referred to the literature.

Finally, one must consider the justification for our particular anatomic approach: the bilateral sectioning of the splanchnic nerves and sympathetic chains supradiaphragmatically. The literature is replete with articles supporting other approaches, specifically unilateral and/or supradiaphragmatic and subdiaphragmatic approaches combined. Some supporters of a unilateral approach have argued that it is sufficient because it has been effective in a small number of cases.[6] Nevertheless, elegant work previously noted has supported bilateral innervation of the pancreas; and cases have been described in which unilateral sympathectomy-splanchnicectomy failed, with relief of symptoms after the second side was ablated.[8] Other unilateral ablative procedures have been shown to be effective initially but with recurrence of pain on the opposite side.[11] The initial success was presumably due to the increase in threshold to painful stimulation that can be achieved in this manner.[1]

The lengths of sympathetic chain and splanchnic nerves resected have varied from a lower thoracic supradiaphragmatic approach[5,10] to a combined lower thoracic and upper lumbar approach from T-7 down to L-2.[2] Once the lumbar ganglia are sacrificed and the more extensively this is done, the greater is the risk of sexual dysfunction.[12] The added subdiaphragmatic approach increases the technical difficulty but has not been shown to increase the frequency or degree of pain relief.

Our preference has been to excise the sympathetic chains and the greater, lesser, and least splanchnic nerves bilaterally from T-9 down to the diaphragm, removing at least three and preferably four ganglia in the process.

RESULTS

Of fifty-six patients with intractable abdominal and/or back pain due to pancreatic carcinoma who underwent bilateral thoracic sympathectomy-splanchnicectomy, 70% had good or complete relief of pain as defined in the study.[10] Fourteen percent of these patients had only slight relief; 16% were complete failures. Twenty-three percent of those with good or complete relief experienced some recurrence or increase in pain, but this was usually with long-term survivors (average 11 months) and was not usually severe. Overall operative mortality in the series of patients subjected to both the ablative neurosurgical procedure and at least a laparotomy was 7%. Failure in some of these patients was explained by involvement of structures innervated by the somatic nervous system (e.g., the anterior abdominal wall) or spread of tumor into the splanchnic nerves and sympathetic chains themselves. The latter situation was present in two of our cases, in one of which there was unrelieved pain after the procedure was performed.

Surgical technique

The patient is placed in the prone position (Fig. 8-1), usually under the same anesthetic as used for the laparotomy. A separate parmedian incision is made on each side, 4 to 5 inches in length and centered over the eleventh rib (Fig. 8-2). The incision measures four fingerbreadths from the midline (Fig. 8-3). After incision through the latissimus dorsi and sacrospinalis, the eleventh rib is exposed with a subperiosteal dissection; a periosteal elevator (Fig. 8-4) and a pigtail dissector are used (Fig. 8-5). The proximal 4 inches of the eleventh rib are resected. Although it is not necessary to disarticulate the head of the rib, it is helpful to make this resection as medial as conveniently possible (Figs. 8-6 to 8-8). Access to the extrapleural space has now been gained, and the exposure is widened with finger dissection (Fig. 8-7) and then maintained by means of a malleable retractor (Fig. 8-8) after the lung has been protected with an appropriately marked sponge.

The ganglionated sympathetic chain is now identified as it runs across the costovertebral articulations, usually just ventral to the head of the rib (Figs. 8-7 to 8-9). This chain is exposed and then is dissected and excised between silver clips from the diaphragm below up to the ninth vertebral ganglion. In so removing the sympathetic chain, the operator resects the white and gray rami communicantes as well as the origins of the least (T-12) and lesser (T-10, T-11) splanchnic nerves (Fig. 8-10) along with some of the connections to the greater splanchnic nerve (T-9) (Fig. 8-11).

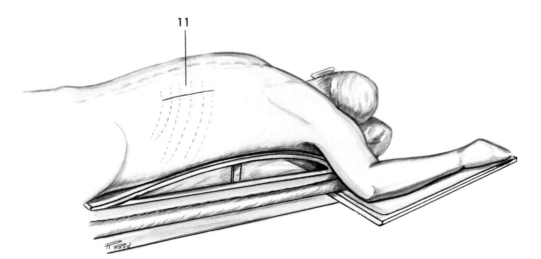

Fig. 8-1. The patient is placed in the prone position on a laminectomy frame, which decreases abdominal pressure and simplifies ventilation. A paramedian incision is shown, approximately 5 inches in length, centered over the eleventh rib and four fingerbreadths from the midline.

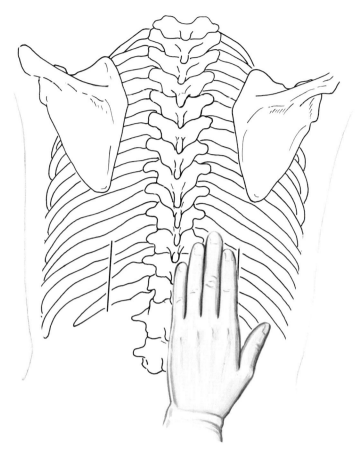

Fig. 8-2. Method used for localizing the skin incision.

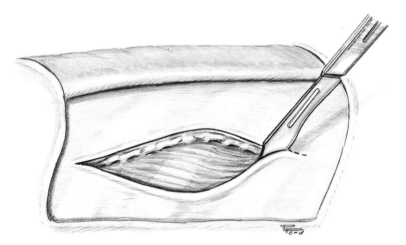

Fig. 8-3. The incision through the skin and subcutaneous tissue is being completed. This allows visualization of the muscles (latissimus dorsi and sacrospinalis) which will be divided to expose the ribs. Cutting cautery is helpful here.

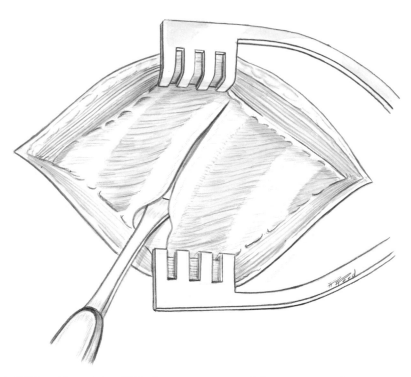

Fig. 8-4. With self-retaining D'Errico retractors used for exposure, the surgeon cuts the periosteum on the dorsal surface of the rib to be removed. A subperiosteal dissection is then completed with a periosteal elevator as shown.

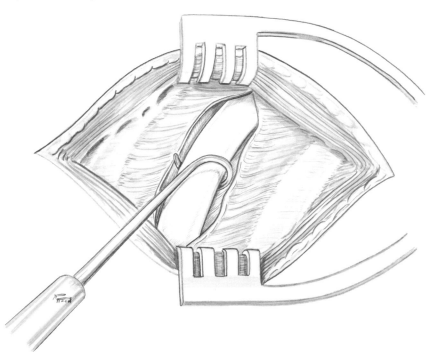

Fig. 8-5. A pigtail-shaped periosteal elevator is used to complete isolation of the rib from the periosteum without endangering the underlying pleura.

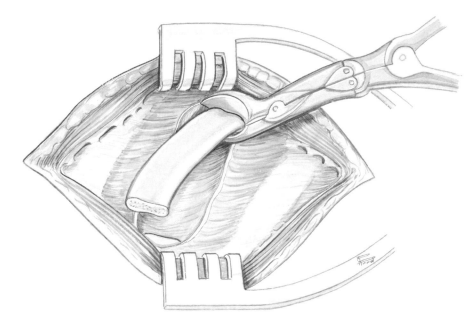

Fig. 8-6. Approximately 4 inches of the isolated eleventh rib are now resected. Although it is not necessary to disarticulate the head of the rib, it is helpful to make this resection as close to the transverse process as conveniently possible to allow adequate exposure.

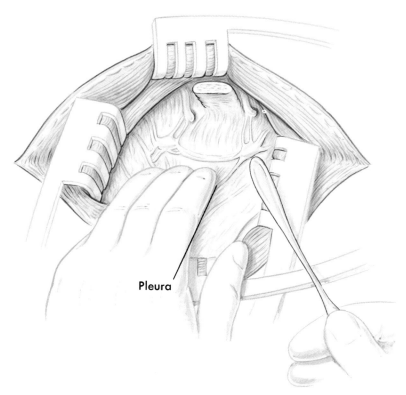

Pleura

Fig. 8-7. Locating the sympathetic chain just ventral to the head of the rib. The surgeon's hand is used, first, for extrapleural blunt dissection of this space and, then, for retraction of the parietal pleura and underlying visceral structures. Exposure can best be maintained by a malleable retractor held by a first assistant. The pleura is protected by a tagged laparotomy sponge.

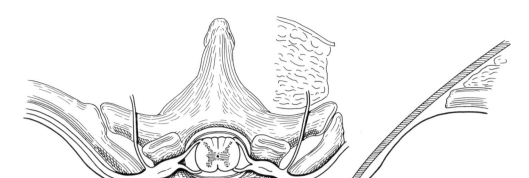

Pleura

Fig. 8-8. Cross section of the view obtained in Fig. 8-7. The sympathetic chain is easily identified with its white and gray rami communicantes leaving and entering the intercostal nerve. Some representative splanchnic nerves have been drawn in cross section, lying in their usual location along the vertebral body. The most important point in this drawing is the presence of a splanchnic nerve running along the parietal pleura and inadvertently covered by the malleable retractor (arrow). One must identify these nerves while dissecting down to the sympathetic chain in the extrapleural space.

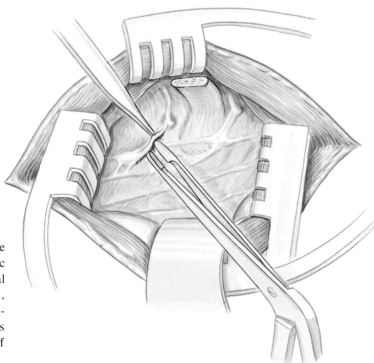

Fig. 8-9. Beginning isolation of the sympathetic chain. The splanchnic nerves are shown along the vertebral body, ventral to the sympathetic chain, and have yet to be isolated. A pistol-grip or bayonet-shaped dissector is helpful in keeping one's hands out of the line of vision.

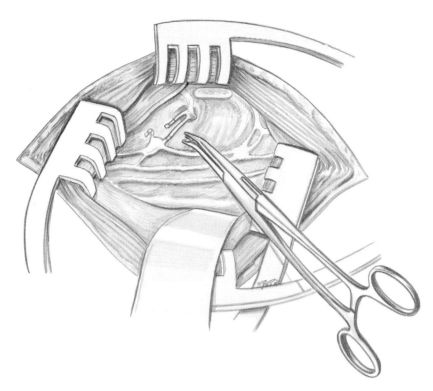

Fig. 8-10. All nerves are sharply incised after either coagulation or clipping with traditional neurosurgical clips. The "silver" clips control small vessel hemorrhage when necessary and provide postoperative roentgenographic verification of the extent of the dissection. Tearing the rami communicantes from the intercostal nerves may lead to neuroma formation and should be avoided.

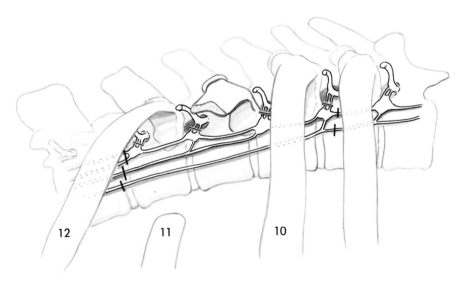

Fig. 8-11. Ideal extent of sympathetic chain removal and splanchnic nerve resection. The short black lines represent silver clips placed during this dissection.

Attention is now turned to removal of the splanchnic nerves along the same extent as the sympathetic chain has been removed. Knowledge of the following points is helpful:

1. The greater splanchnic nerve lies ventral to the sympathetic chain, along the vertebral body. This is a large nerve (origin T-6 through T-9), easily 1.5 to 2.0 mm in diameter, and it must be removed. The smaller nerves identified are the lesser and least splanchnic nerves, often more numerous than anatomically described. The more complete the removal of all these nerves, the more effective will be the procedure.

2. Although typically lying on the vertebral body, the splanchnic nerves, including the greater, may be adherent to the pleura and inadvertently retracted along with the lung (Fig. 8-8, arrow).

3. The greater the length of sympathetic chain and splanchnic nerves resected, the less likely regeneration is to occur.

After removal of the malleable retractor, the wound is "flooded" with sterile irrigation and the lung is held in expansion by the anesthesiologist so pleural tears can be searched for and repaired. The wound is then closed in anatomic layers with 3-0 Neurolon (Fig. 8-12).

An upright chest film is normally taken in the recovery room to look for a pneumothorax, which can be treated by chest tube or observation depending on the percent collapsed.

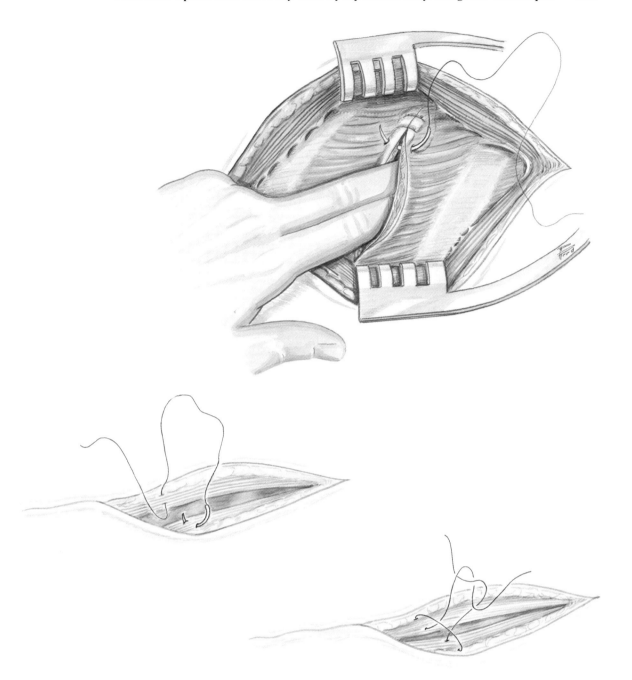

Fig. 8-12. Layer-by-layer reconstitution of the anatomic planes during closure with 3-0 Neurolon. Before the first layer is closed, the extrapleural space is flooded with Ringer's lactate. This will reveal pleural tears which can then be repaired. If a leak is found, a chest tube is placed in the extrapleural space under suction drainage while the layers are closed. When completed, the tube is pulled and the tube site sutured closed.

All patients—with or without leaks—must be followed with postoperative chest roentgenograms in an upright position. Routine postoperative wound care is effected, and the sutures are removed on the sixth postoperative day.

REFERENCES

1. Bingham, J. R., Ingelfinger, F. J., and Smithwick, R. H.: The effects of sympathectomy on abdominal pain in man, Gastroenterology **15:**18, 1950.
2. Connolly, J. E., and Richards, V.: Bilateral splanchnicectomy and lumbodorsal sympathectomy for chronic relapsing pancreatitis, Ann. Surg. **131:**58, 1950.
3. Copping, J., Willix, R., and Kraft, R.: Palliative chemical splanchnicectomy, Arch. Surg. **98:**418, 1969.
4. Gorbitz, C., and Leavens, M. E.: Alcohol block of the celiac plexus for control of upper abdominal pain caused by cancer and pancreatitis, J. Neurosurg. **34:**575, 1971.
5. Heisey, W. G., and Dohn, D. F.: Splanchnicectomy for the treatment of intractable abdominal pain, Cleve. Clin. Q. **34:**9, 1967.
6. Hurwitz, A., and Gurwitz, J.: Relief of pain in chronic relapsing pancreatitis by unilateral sympathectomy, Arch. Surg. **61:**372, 1950.
7. Peet, M. M.: Splanchnic section for hypertension, Univ. Hosp. Bull. Ann Arbor **1:**17, 1935.
8. Ray, B. S., and Neill, C. L.: Abdominal visceral sensation in man, Ann. Surg. **126:**709, 1947.
9. Richin, C. A.: The innervation of the pancreas, J. Comp. Neurol. **83:**223, 1945.
10. Sadar, E. S., and Cooperman, A. M.: Bilateral thoracic sympathectomy-splanchnicectomy in the treatment of intractable pain due to pancreatic carcinoma, Cleve. Clin. Q. **41:**185, 1974.
11. White, J. C.: Choice of surgical procedures for relief of pain in incurable diseases of chest and abdomen, Surg. Clin. North Am. **38:**1373, 1958.
12. Whitelaw, G. P., and Smithwick, R. H.: Some secondary effects of sympathectomy with particular reference to disturbance of sexual function, N. Engl. J. Med. **245:**121, 1951.

CHAPTER 9

Cancer of the pancreatic region

AVRAM M. COOPERMAN
STANLEY O. HOERR

Periampullary carcinoma

Carcinoma of the periampullary region includes *four malignant lesions that arise at or near the ampulla of Vater.* These lesions are in the head of the pancreas, ampulla of Vater, intrapancreatic portion of the common bile duct, and descending portion of the duodenum. Although some reports have included these four lesions in discussions of the results of operative treatment and though the prognosis for the four is limited, the biologic behavior and survival pattern of adenocarcinoma of the head of the pancreas are sufficiently worse than for the other three lesions that there is considerable disagreement about its operative treatment. For this reason two approaches, one aggressive and one conservative, follow. The treatment of carcinoma of the ampulla of Vater, duodenum, and distal common bile duct is less controversial and is discussed briefly.

PREOPERATIVE EVALUATION

The preoperative evaluation of all patients suspected of having a periampullary tumor includes a careful history and physical examination, laboratory tests, and diagnostic roentgenologic procedures. The history, examination, and laboratory tests may suggest only malignant disease and by themselves are not diagnostic. In one large series the bilirubin values ranged from 3 to 35 mg/dl in patients with malignant periampullary lesions.[44] The bilirubin level is dependent on the duration of obstruction and the proximity of the lesion to the common bile duct and will vary for each patient.

153

For all patients with a suspected periampullary lesion, an endoscopic examination of the stomach and duodenum is essential. Encroachment on or invasion of the medial duodenal wall by a pancreatic lesion, an ulcerating duodenal tumor, or a tumor of the ampulla of Vater may be detected and often a biopsy performed preoperatively. This has several advantages. It may establish a definitive diagnosis preoperatively, decrease operating and anesthesia time, and avoid opening of the duodenum at surgery. An upper gastrointestinal series is then done and is of greater help in diagnosing carcinoma of the pancreas than in diagnosing the other three lesions. Widening of the duodenal loop and puckering of the medial duodenal wall are commonly observed. A dilated stomach may indicate impending gastric or duodenal obstruction with any of these lesions.

When the serum bilirubin level precludes an intravenous or oral cholecystogram (it invariably does with these lesions) and the endoscopic examination has not been diagnostic, then percutaneous transhepatic cholangiography (PTHC) or endoscopic retrograde cholangiography (ERC) may locate the level of the obstructing lesion and help establish a diagnosis preoperatively.

These tests are not mutually exclusive and a preference for one must be based on the availability of, experience with, and results achieved by each at a particular institution. A recent randomized prospective study[15] compared both methods in fifty patients. A high degree of diagnostic accuracy was obtained by both, but PTHC had a higher initial positive yield for extrahepatic lesions. We prefer to use endoscopic retrograde studies when the clinical features are atypical and surgery is not clearly indicated and to use "skinny" needle PTHC as a preoperative test performed by our radiologist when extrahepatic causes are suspected.

Selective angiography has been utilized preoperatively[12] to help determine resectability of some lesions and to delineate the pancreatic and hepatic arterial blood supply that may be anomalous. Although occasionally we utilize preoperative angiography, surgery is almost always indicated to relieve biliary and/or gastric obstruction. Thus accurate determination of resectability and delineation of anatomy can be made at operation and angiography is optional.

PANCREATIC RESECTION

History. The early history of pancreatic surgery has been summarized by Warren and co-workers.[44] In the United States in 1898, Halsted[21] performed a segmental resection of the descending duodenum with implantation of the common bile and pancreatic ducts. The operation was performed for an ampullary cancer, and the patient died 7 months later of recurrent tumor.

Because resections of the head of the pancreas were thought to be incompatible with life, resections were done for ampullary, ductal, or duodenal cancers and consisted of duodenal resections, sparing the head of the pancreas.

In 1941 Hunt[26] summarized fifty-nine ampullary cancers, fifty-three of which had been excised by local treatment (operative mortality, 44%). Six patients survived more than a year, one of whom, operated on in 1910, lived nine years after transduodenal excision.

In 1935 Whipple, Parsons, and Mullins[48] reported an operation that bears the name of the senior surgeon. This was done in two stages. At the first operation a cholecystogastrostomy (now obsolete) was done and the distal common bile duct ligated and divided. At the second stage the duodenum between the pylorus and its ascending portion and a wedge of the head of the pancreas was excised. The pancreas was reapproximated, the distal duodenum and pylorus oversewn, and a side-to-side gastrojejunostomy made.

Two years later, on February 11, 1937, Brunschwig[7] performed a pancreaticoduodenal resection for a large cancer of the head of the pancreas in two stages. The distal stomach was resected, and the pancreas to the right of the superior mesenteric vein was excised. The transected pancreas was then oversewn. The patient survived the operation but died of widespread metastases on April 26, 1937. In 1945 Whipple[47] reported a five-year survival after a one-stage resection for an islet cell tumor.

Although one-stage resections are done today, a number of postoperative deaths have been attributed to hepatic or renal failure. These complications usually develop in jaundiced patients whose bilirubin is higher than 30 mg/dl or whose jaundice has been present for months. A preliminary biliary decompression is worthwhile in these circumstances.[1,4]

MALIGNANT DISEASE PRODUCING JAUNDICE

Jaundice may be a presenting manifestation of malignant periampullary lesions from four different anatomic origins: (1) head of the pancreas, by far the most common (and with the worst prognosis), (2) ampulla of Vater (the best prognosis), (3) descending duodenum, and (4) distal common bile duct.

The decision to explore the patient presumed to have obstructive jaundice will not be influenced by the source of the obstruction. Proof that the obstruction is malignant must often await assessment at operation. Similarly the procedure to be performed, whether curative or palliative, will depend more on the extent of regional involvement by the primary lesion and the presence or absence of regional or distant metastases than on the site of origin.

HEAD OF THE PANCREAS

Natural history. Of 100 patients with adenocarcinoma of the head of the pancreas who undergo surgery, 70% have disseminated disease, 20% have regional nodes involved, and 5% to 10% have localized tumors at the time of diagnosis.[2] Thus the *possible number* of resectable adenocarcinomas is low. The fact that the survival is poor for all patients has been shown in two extensive reviews in which the overall one-year and three-year survivals were 7.6% and 1.2% regardless of treatment.[2,40]

When subdivisions based on local, regional, and disseminated disease are evaluated, survival patterns are still very poor. At 12 months after diagnosis, 4% of patients with disseminated disease, 18% with regional disease, and 20% with local disease will be alive. At 30 months 0% to 15% with disseminated disease, 3% with regional nodes, and 5% with local disease will be alive; and at 60 months less than 2% of patients with regional or local disease will survive.[2,14] Some patients without biopsy and a bypass will survive five years and more because the disease was not cancer but pancreatitis or because the tumor was less aggressive.

Preresection biopsy. Many surgeons subscribe to the belief that a positive biopsy for malignant disease should be obtained before a patient is subjected to the hazards of a pancreaticoduodenal resection. However, successful biopsy may be quite difficult in patients with a suspected periampullary lesion and a mass in the head of the pancreas. In roughly 50% the biopsy, irrespective of technique, will fail to yield tissue on which the pathologist can make a positive diagnosis of cancer by frozen section. Needle aspiration biopsy is probably the simplest and safest method and is acquiring a reputation for accuracy, but it requires experience both in using the technique and in interpreting the tissue.

We have adopted in recent years a more liberal attitude, considering all the available evidence and employing knowledgeable consultation in the operating room. A blind resection (i.e., without positive pathologic evidence for cancer) seems justified for small lesions producing jaundice in good-risk patients with a compatible history for malignant obstruction and with concurrence by one or more experienced consultants who scrub up and palpate the lesion. Such intraoperative consultation may sway the decision in either direction. It also has the advantage of permitting several surgeons to acquire experience from a single patient in these comparatively rare surgical problems.

One of us (S.O.H.) in an experience of twenty-four years and 125 patients performed pancreatic resection for attempted cure in only six patients (5%); two of these operations were total pancreatectomy. There were no operative deaths, and five of the patients died within two years; only the remaining patient—one of the 125—was a possible five-year survivor after resection.

Does cell type influence prognosis? Since 90% of pancreatic tumors and carcinomas arise from ductal or acinar epithelium, less than 10% of patients have other potentially more favorable lesions. The prognosis for islet cell tumors, papillary tumors, and cystadenomas is better than for ductal adenocarcinomas.[2] The best prognosis is for islet cell tumors.

In the review by Baylor and Berg,[2] 17% of islet cell tumors were apparently localized to the pancreas at the time of diagnosis. Even when islet cell tumors have local and disseminated metastases, survival at 4 years has been 60% and 18% respectively. Unfortunately this tumor is rare, being encountered in less than 2% of cases.

Does sex or age influence survival? End results do not seem to be statistically altered by sex or age, though the prognosis may be worse in older patients (past 65 years).[2]

Therapeutic alternatives. When the cancer is clearly incurable by reason of local extension or distant metastases, only palliation is possible by surgical means. Palliative procedures are discussed separately.[16,52]

If the lesion is small and apparently localized, it is potentially and theoretically curable by resection. Pancreaticoduodenectomy is a formidable operation with a variable mortality.* A mortality rate less than 10% is reported by the most accomplished surgeons. A resection, even if cure seems possible, may be poor judgment in a patient who is in poor physical condition.

If the patient is not a prohibitive surgical risk, there are still two schools of thought as to what course should be followed. Many surgeons favor an attempt at curative resection using either (1) the standard pancreaticoduodenectomy (the Whipple operation)† or (2) total pancreatectomy in view of a reported 30% incidence of multicentricity of the tumor and to eliminate the hazard of leakage from the pancreaticojejunal anastomosis.[23,37a,39] A third alternative, extended total pancreatectomy, which includes resection of the superior mesenteric artery and portal vein, has a high operative mortality with a yet unproved benefit.[17] Extensive resections, including segments of portal or mesenteric veins, have been reported but though technically possible did not prolong life.[11,25,32]

A sharply divergent view is advocated by George Crile, Jr.,[14] of the Cleveland Clinic, who for cancer of the head of the pancreas favors biliary bypass (accompanied by gastroenteric bypass if indicated) on the grounds that the risk of a resection outweighs the chance of cure and bypass offers better palliation when resection fails to cure.

Analysis of published reports. It is difficult to analyze and interpret published reports because of study designs that are not comparable, lack of follow-up, absence of randomization, and (to begin with) the very

*References 3, 8, 20, 22, 23, 30, 33, 35, 36, 40, 49.
†References 5, 8, 16, 22, 24, 29, 30, 33.

limited curability of these lesions. Satisfactory prospective randomized studies are probably not in the realm of practicability, particularly as they relate to procedures designed to cure, if only because of the infrequency of potentially curable lesions in the head of the pancreas. Unfortunately most lesions are clearly incurable at the time of exploration because of fixation to surrounding structures, the presence of regional or distant metastases, or both.

Operative mortality in the published series of pancreatic resections for cancer varies from 8% to 44%,* and five-year survivals from 0% to 12%.[2,34] Nakase and co-workers[37] reviewed 3,610 patients with periampullary cancer treated in fifty-seven Japanese institutions. The operative mortality following pancreatic resection was 25.3%, and six of 230 survivors or 3% survived five years (histologic type not specified). A morbidity rate at least equal to the mortality rate also occurs. In seventeen series comprising 496 cases of cancer of the head of the pancreas,[40] after pancreatic resection 4% of the patients lived five years. The mean operative mortality was 21%, and the mean postoperative survival 14 months. Although survival is usually longer in patients who have had resection as opposed to bypass, in most series the groups are not comparable. The patients with advanced disease are usually the poorest risks and have been relegated to the bypass groups.

A further claim made for pancreatic resection is that as a palliative procedure it is better than bypass.[33] Less pain and a better state of health have followed this procedure. However, resection has not been compared to pain-ablating procedures like splanchnic resection or injection; and the value of the larger procedure for pain relief is not known. Certainly the risk of resection exceeds that of splanchnic injection.

Conclusions. The procedure to be performed will naturally depend on a number of factors, including age of the patient, coexistence of serious medical diseases, technical problems presented by the lesion, and the surgeon's philosophy or past experiences.

If resection is decided on, most surgeons will probably perform the standard pancreaticoduodenectomy for small lesions in good-risk young patients and avoid total pancreatectomy (unless the remaining pancreas is unsuitable for anastomosis), preferring the theoretical chance of multicentricity to the certainty of establishing surgical insulin dependence and pancreatic insufficiency. The ideal patient for resection would be a young previously healthy individual with a small islet cell tumor localized in the head of the gland.

If the patient is a poor risk or has proved regional metastases, with even small lesions, the simpler safer palliative procedures will probably be

*References 1, 3, 8, 18, 19, 22, 24, 29, 30, 33, 35.

a wiser choice, including the possible use of splanchnicectomy for control of pain.

AMPULLA OF VATER AND PERIAMPULLARY REGION

Tumors in this region are characteristically small and usually papillary at the time they obstruct the common bile duct, and diagnosis is thus possible at a relatively early stage (Figs. 9-1 and 9-2). The result is surgical exploration when a resection for cure can be attempted in more than half the cases. In a recent review of our experience with thirty eight ampullary

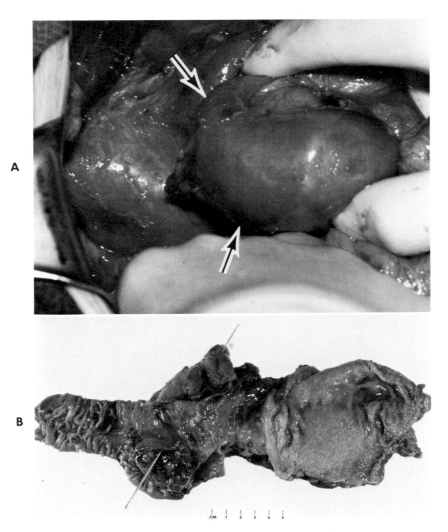

Fig. 9-1. A, Large papillary exophytic cancer of the ampulla of Vater seen through the duodenal wall. The duodenum has been mobilized by incising the lateral peritoneal reflection. Arrows outline the extent of the tumor. **B,** Specimen after pancreaticoduodenostomy. The probe is through the common bile duct.

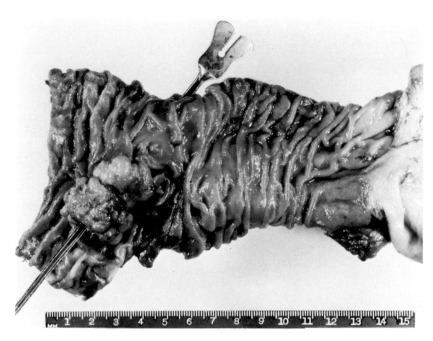

Fig. 9-2. Large exophytic papillary adenocarcinoma of the ampulla of Vater. After a pancreaticoduodenal resection the patient lived fifteen years before he died of a myocardial infarct.

Table 9-1. Cancer of the ampulla of Vater: results of operative treatment in thirty-eight patients

	Pancreaticoduodenectomy	Bypass	Bypass and excision
Number of patients	23	7	8
Number alive	9*	1	1
Number dead	14	6	7
Time since operation (mo)	7,12,18†,24,44, 131,216	30	34
Operative mortality	2(9%)	1(14%)	1(13%)
Dead of metastases	10	5	5
Time (mo) from surgery to death	15,15,16,18,24,30, 33,36,36,38,78	6,11,23,24,54	3,24,24,42,72
Mean time (mo)	29	23	——

*Two lost to follow-up at 29 and 72 months.
†One patient had recurrence 12 months postoperatively.

tumors,[31] the lesion appeared to be surgically curable by resection in twenty-three patients at the time of exploration (Table 9-1).

Therapeutic alternatives

For cure:

1. A pancreaticoduodenal resection
2. Excision (or electrocautery destruction) of the ampullary tumor with or without biliary enteric bypass

For palliation or as a first stage in anticipation of a curative second stage operation:

3. Biliary enteric bypass (cholecystoenterostomy or choledochoenterostomy)

Analysis of published reports. Since all reviews of treatment of ampullary cancer are retrospective, the limitations of comparing different operations are obvious.

As with cancer of the head of the pancreas, the more favorable lesions and younger healthier patients generally undergo pancreaticoduodenal resection whereas bypass operations are reserved for unfavorable lesions or patients with coexisting serious medical diseases or anticipated limited survival. Differences in survival between operations may reflect case selection rather than the operation per se. The prognosis for exophytic papillary lesions of the ampulla is at least twice as good as that for ulcerating and infiltrating lesions.[31]

Pancreaticoduodenal resection. This procedure should offer the best chance of cure for ampullary cancers because it is the only operation that widely removes tumor and surrounding tissue.

Despite the theoretical advantages of this operation, the long-term survivors are usually patients who have a papillary noninfiltrating cancer with negative nodes. Warren and co-workers[45] reported five-year and ten-year survival rates of 40% and 35% after pancreaticoduodenectomy when nodes were negative but only 9% when regional nodes were metastatically involved. We noted that only four of twenty-three patients survived five years after pancreaticoduodenal resection, two of whom are living at eleven and eighteen years postoperatively.[31] Nakase and co-workers[37] reported that seventeen of 285 patients (6%) survived five years and seven (3%) survived ten years. Our mean survival after pancreaticoduodenal resection was 55 months when nodes were negative and 23 months when nodes were positive. Thus realization of cure occurred in four of twenty-three attempts and the cause of death in nearly all patients was metastasis.

Bypass with excision of the ampulla. Eight of our patients underwent this operation. Six have died of metastases (mean survival, 25 months). One patient is alive at 34 months. Wise and co-workers[50] reported a five-year survival of 38% in twenty-eight patients after local excision of the ampullary tumor. They referred to a literature review of 123 patients with ampullary cancer thirty-seven of whom survived two to twenty-two years following excision of the ampullary tumor. Our results are not comparable since these patients were either elderly or had metastatic disease or other competing illnesses at the time of surgery.

Bypass alone. Of seven patients who underwent bypass procedures alone (cholecysto- or choledochoenteric bypass), survival was similar to that of patients who underwent bypass plus excision of the ampulla (mean, 23 months).

Conclusions. Regardless of the operation performed, it is clear that late deaths from ampullary carcinomas large or small are nearly always due to metastatic disease. If regional nodes are involved, the five-year survival rate is reduced by half to two thirds. The survival is twice as good for papillary as for infiltrating lesions.

Although the opposing philosophies regarding curative resection referred to in the discussion of carcinoma of the head of the pancreas can apply here, the data are even more difficult to analyze since young healthy patients with favorable tumors almost always undergo resection. The fact that some of these tumors are potentially curable has provided encouragement for surgeons to attempt resection, though the actual number of long-term survivors is low. From a practical standpoint in patients with ampullary cancer without regional metastases, a pancreaticoduodenectomy may be undertaken with the attempt to cure. When regional nodes are involved by tumor, evidence supporting resection is less clear and the competing risks must be carefully assessed.

EXTRAHEPATIC BILE DUCTS

Life expectancy for patients who have cancer of the extrahepatic bile ducts (Fig. 9-3) is limited. Compared with that for patients who have pancreatic cancer, the outlook is excellent; but the comparison is relative. The most optimistic reports show a five-year survival in patients undergoing resection of no more (and usually less) than 40%.[5,43,45]

Since these lesions can occur in the upper, middle, or lower common bile duct, the lower duct lesions are often not separated from the more proximal lesions. In two large series totalling more than 250 patients with bile duct cancers, only thirty patients had tumors of the distal third of the common bile duct. Thus large numbers of patients are not available for analyses.[5,34] Nakase and co-workers[37] reported 132 resections for terminal bile duct cancers; six patients (5%) survived five years, and one (1%) lived ten years.

Limited survival of patients with a bile duct cancer has been attributed to (1) the presence of distant metastases at the initial operation (in at least

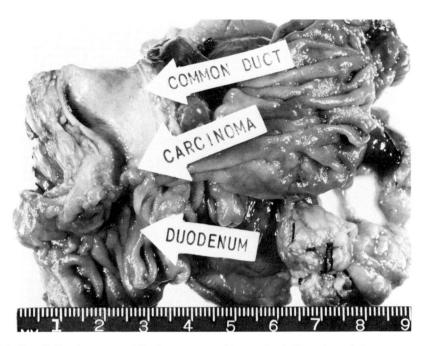

Fig. 9-3. Small distal common bile duct tumor with proximal dilatation of the common duct. The patient underwent pancreaticoduodenal resection.

33%), (2) perineural invasion (in 66%), and (3) extraductal metastases (in 30% to 50%).[5,42]

Of 173 Lahey Clinic patients with a bile duct cancer (at all levels of the duct), only twenty five survived treatment one or more years, 42% died within a month of treatment, and 103 (60%) died within 6 months of treatment.[5]

From a practical standpoint, it is frequently difficult clinically to separate lower bile duct cancers from ampullary or other periampullary lesions. Even in experienced hands, misdiagnosis at surgery occurs at least 10% of the time.[43] When this occurs, treatment is dictated mainly by the local operative findings. When the lesion is confined to the lower third of the duct and does not have associated metastases, an attempt at curative resection can be made. When lymph nodes are metastatically involved, survival is probably limited and the operative risk of resection must be weighed against the chance of prolonged survival.

DUODENUM

Malignant tumors of the duodenum are fortunately uncommon, for despite treatment their outlook is uniformly poor. It has been estimated that 3% of all gastrointestinal cancers occur in the small intestine, and nearly half of these are in the duodenum. As early as 1916, Jefferson[27] noted that, "considering the shortness of the duodenum, it is evident that inch for inch it is more liable to cancer than the rest of the small intestine."

Nearly half these malignant lesions are carcinoma, and the remainder are leiomyosarcoma or lymphosarcoma.[10,28] It is sometimes difficult also to separate these tumors from other periampullary tumors. The symptoms depend on tumor size and proximity to the pylorus and ampulla. Obstruction of the duodenum or ampulla and invasion or ulceration of the duodenal wall produce the symptoms. Approximately 50% of patients are jaundiced (much less than with other periampullary lesions).[10]

Treatment. Surgical treatment will be dictated by the type and location of the tumor and the local and regional findings.

A review of our recent experience (sixteen patients treated at the Cleveland Clinic, 1955 through 1975) emphasizes the aggressive behavior of this lesion and the limited outlook despite treatment methods[13]:

1. Thirteen had a carcinoma.
2. One had a rhabdomyosarcoma.
3. Two had a leiomyosarcoma.

The latter three patients were moribund at the time of examination and no surgery could be done.

Three operations were performed: (1) a pancreaticoduodenal resection (Whipple operation) in six patients, (2) a gastrojejunostomy in three patients, and (3) a segmental resection of the tumor or duodenum with end-to-end duodenoduodenostomy or duodenojejunostomy in four patients (Table 9-2).

Of the thirteen patients who underwent surgery, three are alive. Five of the six pancreaticoduodenal resection patients died of metastases 6 to 61 months after the operation (only one lived five years). The one remaining survivor is alive 26 months after surgery. All three bypass

Table 9-2. Duodenal cancer: results of operative treatment in thirteen patients

	Pancreaticoduodenal resection	Bypass	Segmental resection
Number of patients	6	3	4
Number alive	1 (26 mo)	0	2 (21 and 22 yr)
Number dead	5	3	2
Dead of metastases	6 mo	11 mo	26 mo
	19 mo	14 mo	8½ yr
	26 mo	30 mo	
	30 mo		
	61 mo		

patients died after gastrojejunostomy at 11 to 30 months. Two patients with a tumor in the third portion of the duodenum survive twenty-one and twenty-two years after resection (one after wedge excision of a leiomyosarcoma, the second after duodenal resection with end-to-end anastomosis for adenocarcinoma).

This survival pattern is similar to the survival pattern in other series, in which the follow-up period is often shorter, though five-year survivals of 40% have been reported by some authors.[45] Our approach as guided by these data is (1) to do and advocate segmental resections of the duodenum for adenocarcinoma of the third and fourth portions, (2) to do a wedge excision or segmental resection for leiomyosarcoma that does not approximate the ampulla, and (3) to reserve and employ pancreaticoduodenal resection for adenocarcinoma involving the periampullary areas when metastases are not present. This operation is done only with the hope of cure

BODY AND TAIL OF THE PANCREAS

Certainly the most dismal of all pancreatic neoplasms is adenocarcinoma arising in the body and tail of the gland. The occasional long-term survivors have been patients whose tumor was discovered serendipitously at surgery done for other reasons (Fig. 9-4). Two reports, one by Glenn and

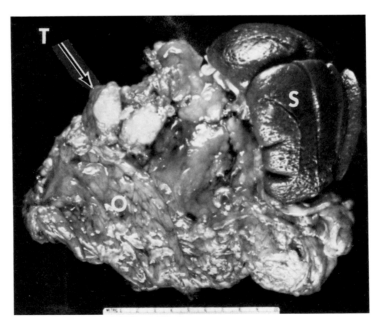

Fig. 9-4. Adenocarcinoma of the body of the pancreas (angioinvasive). The spleen *(S)*, omentum *(O)*, and tumor *(T, arrow)* are shown. This lesion was discovered at the time a 9 kg benign ovarian cyst was excised. The patient is alive six years postoperatively.

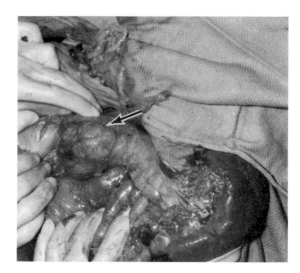

Fig. 9-5. Large nonfunctioning islet cell tumor (arrow) of the body of the pancreas. Distal resection with splenectomy is the treatment of choice.

Thorbjarnarson[19] (five patients) and the second by Warren[43] (ten patients), support this statement; all patients died within two years following resection. At the Cleveland Clinic no adenocarcinoma of the body or tail of the pancreas suspected or diagnosed preoperatively has been resectable, and the sole long-term survivor is a patient whose tumor was discovered at the time of splenectomy. One other patient had an adenocarcinoma (with angioinvasion) resected six years previously (at the Mayo Clinic by A.M.C.) and is free of disease at present (Fig. 9-4). The prognosis is better with islet cell tumors of the body of the pancreas, particularly when resectable (Fig. 9-5).

Since the presenting symptom of most cancers of the body and tail is pain, an abdominal operation is usually combined with a pain-relieving procedure (e.g., splanchnic resection or alcohol injection of the splanchnic plexus). Recently laparotomy has been avoided in a few patients by percutaneous biopsy guided by angiography, computed tomography, or laparoscopy.

Surgical technique (Whipple)

Pancreaticoduodenal resection

This operation is divided into three phases:
1. Determining resectability (Figs. 9-6 to 9-17)
2. Resection (Figs. 9-18 to 9-25)
3. Reconstruction (Figs. 9-26 to 9-32)

DETERMINING RESECTABILITY

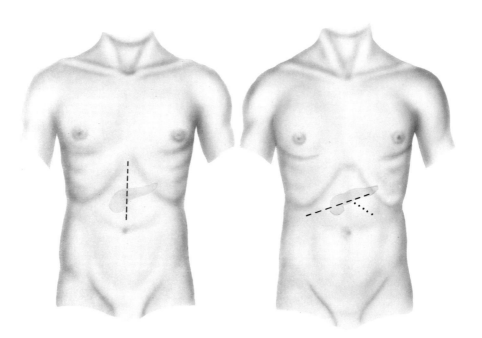

Fig. 9-6. Three incisions commonly used for pancreaticoduodenal resection. Most often the upper midline incision is used. The right upper abdominal oblique or subcostal incision is used for obese patients or when a wide costal arch is present; it may be enlarged to the left as shown by the dotted line.

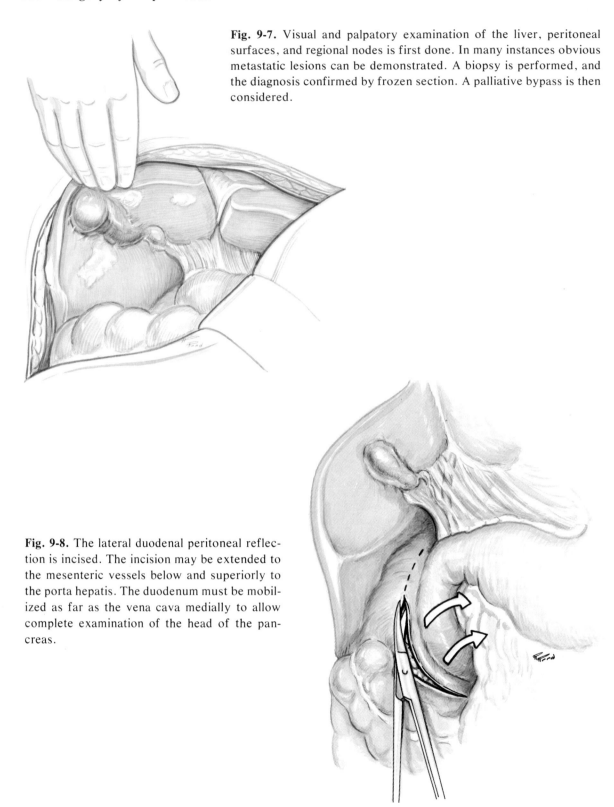

Fig. 9-7. Visual and palpatory examination of the liver, peritoneal surfaces, and regional nodes is first done. In many instances obvious metastatic lesions can be demonstrated. A biopsy is performed, and the diagnosis confirmed by frozen section. A palliative bypass is then considered.

Fig. 9-8. The lateral duodenal peritoneal reflection is incised. The incision may be extended to the mesenteric vessels below and superiorly to the porta hepatis. The duodenum must be mobilized as far as the vena cava medially to allow complete examination of the head of the pancreas.

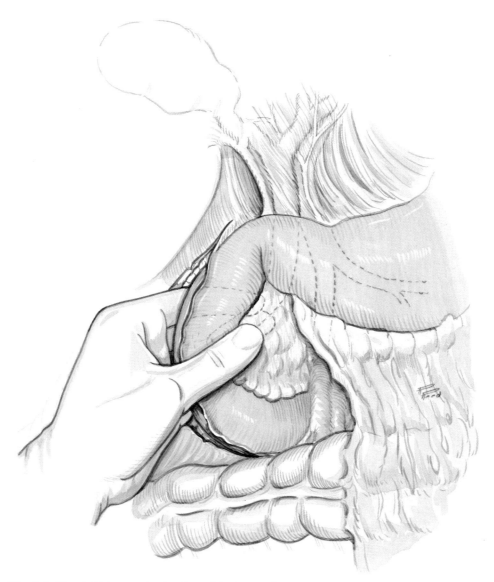

Fig. 9-9. Careful bimanual palpation of the head of the pancreas is next done. In this patient a small cancer of the ampulla was found.

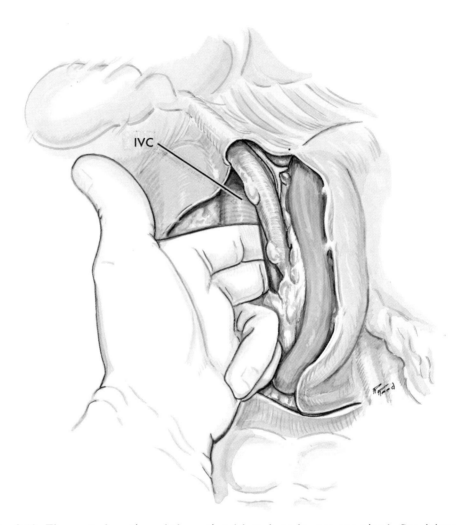

Fig. 9-10. The porta hepatis and the regional lymph nodes are examined. Suspicious or enlarged nodes are removed for frozen section examination. Many surgeons regard a metastatic node as evidence of incurability. A dilated common bile duct secondary to an ampullary tumor is illustrated. *IVC,* Inferior vena cava.

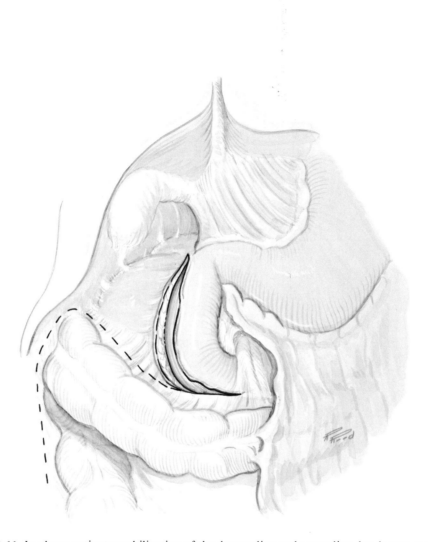

Fig. 9-11. In obese patients mobilization of the descending and ascending duodenum may be difficult. The surgeon mobilizes the ascending and right transverse colon by incising the peritoneal reflection around the colon. Downward traction will allow visualization and exposure of the mesenteric vessels.

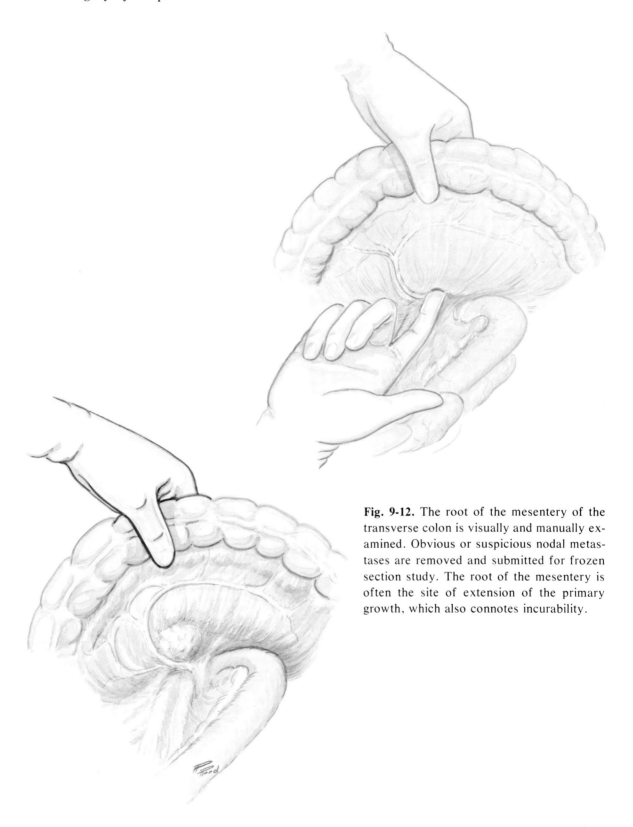

Fig. 9-12. The root of the mesentery of the transverse colon is visually and manually examined. Obvious or suspicious nodal metastases are removed and submitted for frozen section study. The root of the mesentery is often the site of extension of the primary growth, which also connotes incurability.

Fig. 9-13. The fourth portion of the duodenum may be mobilized beneath the mesenteric vessels by incision of the duodenojejunal ligament (superior to the mesocolon) or if more convenient the ligament of Treitz beneath the mesocolon (as shown here).

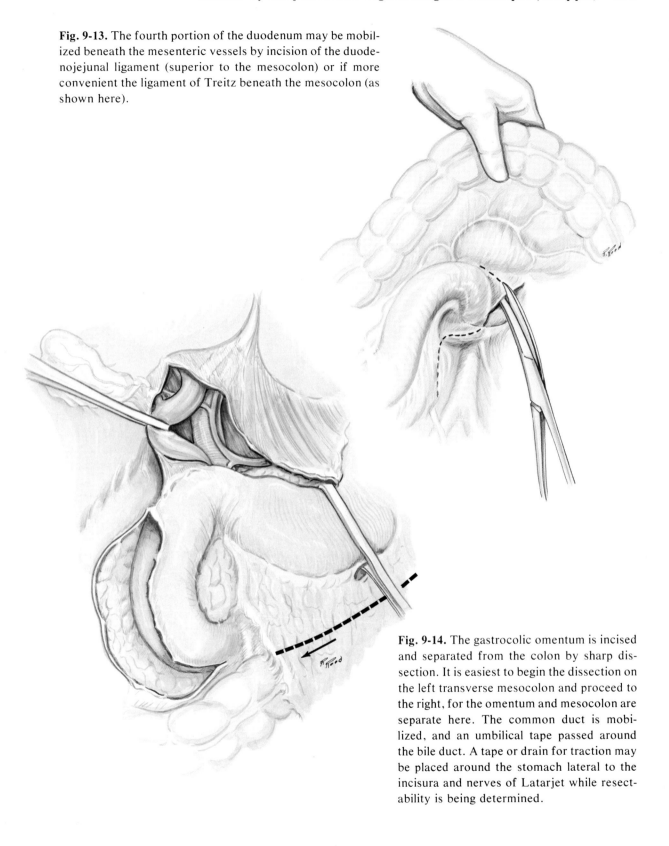

Fig. 9-14. The gastrocolic omentum is incised and separated from the colon by sharp dissection. It is easiest to begin the dissection on the left transverse mesocolon and proceed to the right, for the omentum and mesocolon are separate here. The common duct is mobilized, and an umbilical tape passed around the bile duct. A tape or drain for traction may be placed around the stomach lateral to the incisura and nerves of Latarjet while resectability is being determined.

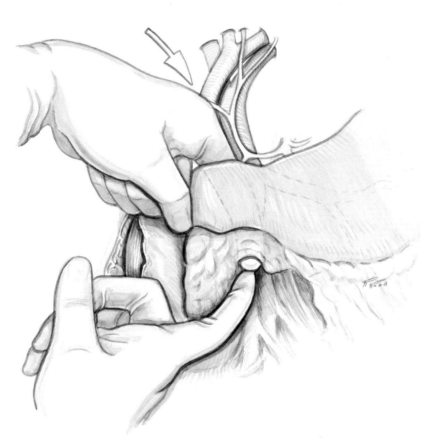

Fig. 9-15. A crucial maneuver to determine resectability is whether the portal vein is mobile and free from the surrounding pancreas. The surgeon inserts his left index finger between the portal vein and the pancreas. His right index finger may be placed on the anterior surface of the mesenteric vein below to meet the advancing left finger. This plane is dissected bluntly.

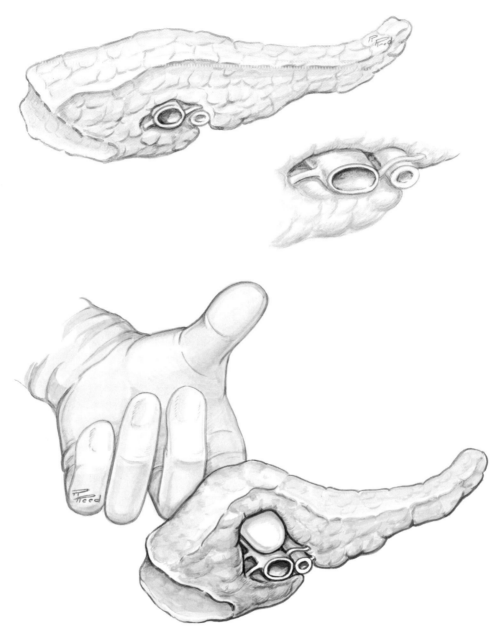

Fig. 9-16. Relationship of the pancreas to the superior mesenteric vein in cross section. The vessels from the uncinate process enter the vein on the right lateral side. The ventral surface is free and the dissection should be carried on this surface.

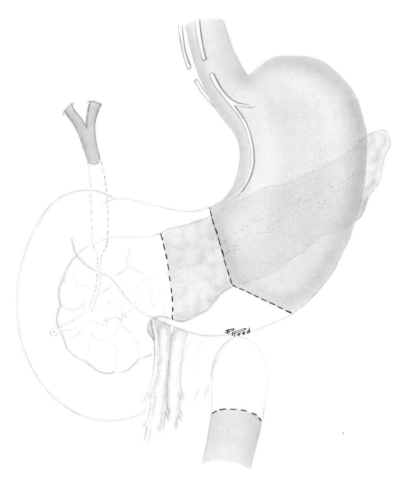

Fig. 9-17. If the portal vein is free of tumor extension, resection for possible cure may be undertaken. The shaded areas are the portions of stomach, bile duct, and jejunum that will remain after resection. The unshaded areas represent the resected specimen. We usually add truncal or selective vagotomy rather than high resection.

RESECTION

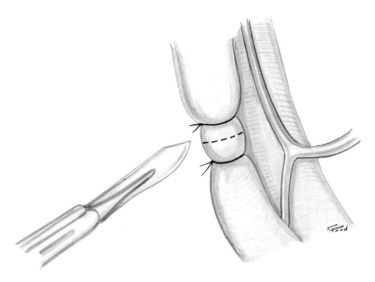

Fig. 9-18. The common bile duct is ligated and divided between ties (to prevent bile leak).

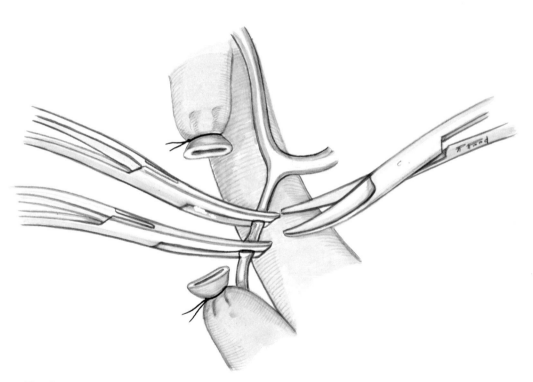

Fig. 9-19. The gastroduodenal artery is ligated near its origin from the hepatic artery and divided. The junction with the hepatic artery should be accurately visualized to preclude accidental ligation of the hepatic artery.

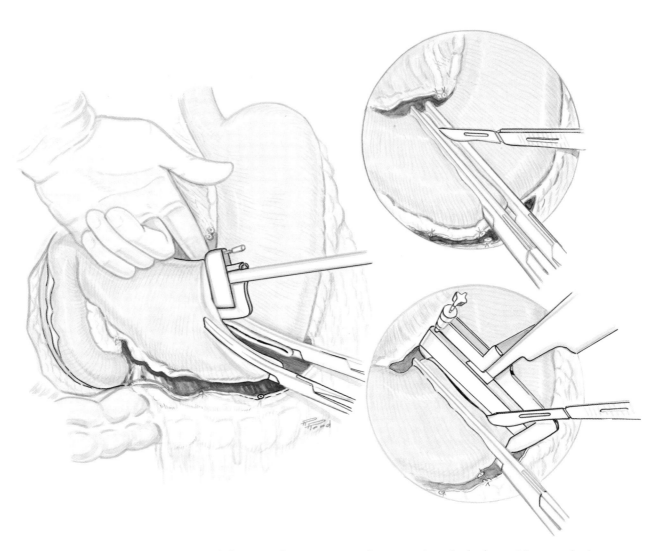

Fig. 9-20. Then it is convenient to transect the stomach at the incisura. Many methods are employed for this. Three are shown here. I (A.M.C.) prefer to use a noncrushing clamp on the greater curvature and a stapler on the lesser curvature.

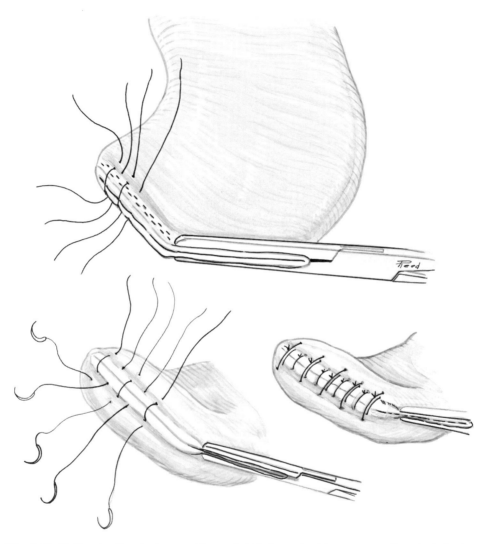

Fig. 9-21. If the stapling instrument is used, it is important to oversew the stapled edges, since hemostasis may not otherwise be secure.

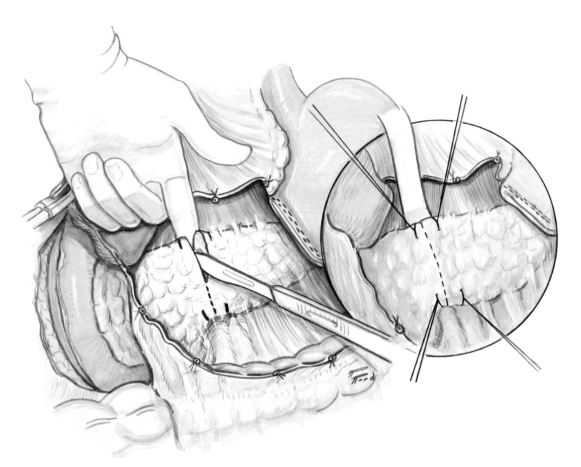

Fig. 9-22. Before transecting pancreas, the surgeon places four traction sutures or large hemoclips on the upper and lower borders of the gland. This helps control bleeding from the transverse pancreatic vessels. Overlapping mattress sutures near the line of resection are another means of ensuring hemostasis. He then divides the pancreas. To further protect the superior mesenteric vein from injury, he may divide the gland over a finger, a malleable retractor, or a clamp. Should the wrong tissue plane be entered and venous bleeding develop, a small pack placed alongside the mesenteric vein will control bleeding from the uncinate branches. If the mesenteric vein is injured, the surgeon can facilitate direct repair by dividing the pancreas, permitting exposure of the entire anterior and lateral surface of the mesenteric vein.

Although nonfatal ligation of the portal vein has been reported,[11] it is hazardous. In the rare circumstance when it must be contemplated, improved exposure and length of the mesenteric vein can be accomplished by mobilizing the root of the mesentery and hepatic and splenic flexures. An additional alternative is to use the splenic vein swung down to the distal mesenteric vein (not shown). A noncrushing clamp may be placed across distal pancreas for better hemostasis.

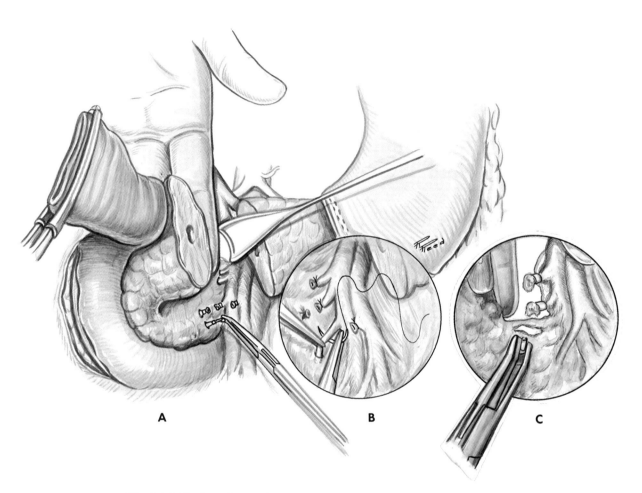

A   **B**   **C**

Fig. 9-23. To free the uncinate process from the mesenteric vein, the surgeon retracts the head of the pancreas to the patient's right and the mesenteric vein gently to the left. A vein retractor is useful here. The vessels from the uncinate process are then identified. They may be divided between hemoclips (**A**) or sutures (**B**). When inflammation obscures these vessels (**C**), we prefer to leave behind some of the uncinate process, dividing it between large hemoclips placed parallel with the mesenteric vein. This is a safer method, and there is much less bleeding.

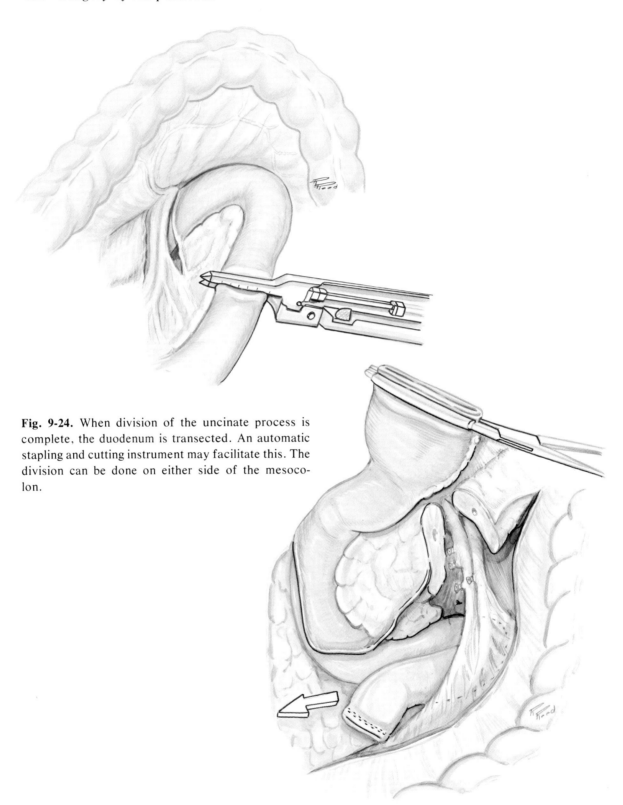

Fig. 9-24. When division of the uncinate process is complete, the duodenum is transected. An automatic stapling and cutting instrument may facilitate this. The division can be done on either side of the mesocolon.

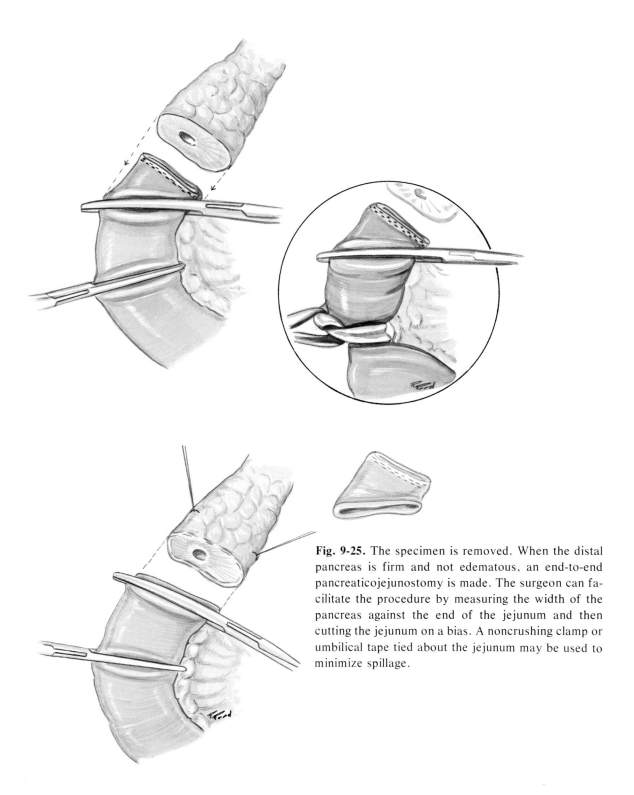

Fig. 9-25. The specimen is removed. When the distal pancreas is firm and not edematous, an end-to-end pancreaticojejunostomy is made. The surgeon can facilitate the procedure by measuring the width of the pancreas against the end of the jejunum and then cutting the jejunum on a bias. A noncrushing clamp or umbilical tape tied about the jejunum may be used to minimize spillage.

RECONSTRUCTION

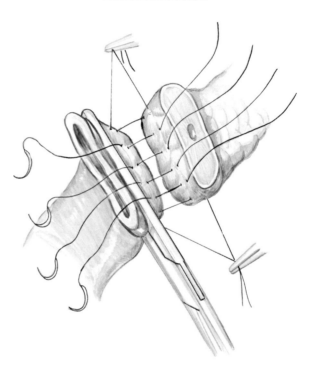

Fig. 9-26. Interrupted nonabsorbable sutures of 3-0 or 4-0 silk are placed between the jejunum and posterior pancreas and are tied.

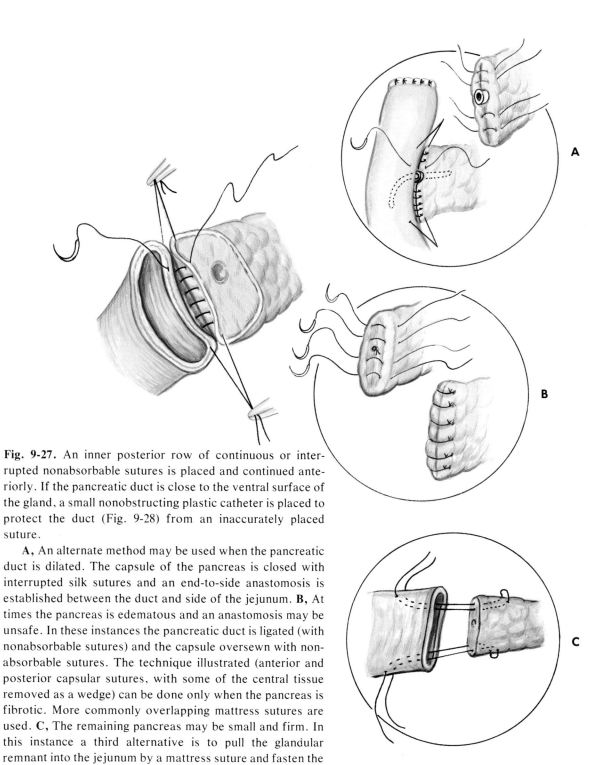

Fig. 9-27. An inner posterior row of continuous or interrupted nonabsorbable sutures is placed and continued anteriorly. If the pancreatic duct is close to the ventral surface of the gland, a small nonobstructing plastic catheter is placed to protect the duct (Fig. 9-28) from an inaccurately placed suture.

A, An alternate method may be used when the pancreatic duct is dilated. The capsule of the pancreas is closed with interrupted silk sutures and an end-to-side anastomosis is established between the duct and side of the jejunum. **B,** At times the pancreas is edematous and an anastomosis may be unsafe. In these instances the pancreatic duct is ligated (with nonabsorbable sutures) and the capsule oversewn with nonabsorbable sutures. The technique illustrated (anterior and posterior capsular sutures, with some of the central tissue removed as a wedge) can be done only when the pancreas is fibrotic. More commonly overlapping mattress sutures are used. **C,** The remaining pancreas may be small and firm. In this instance a third alternative is to pull the glandular remnant into the jejunum by a mattress suture and fasten the capsule to jejunum.

A fourth alternative, pancreaticogastrostomy,[30a] has been used. We have had limited experience with this technique, but its advocates have found it safe and easy to perform.

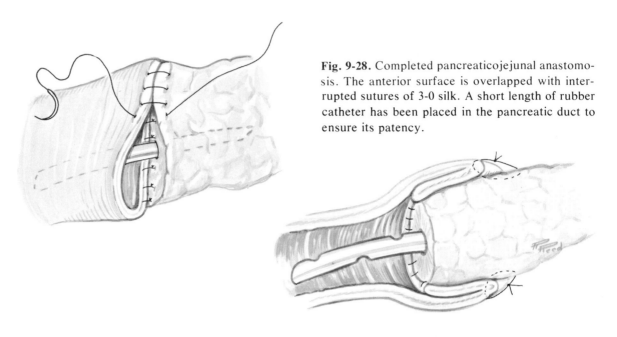

Fig. 9-28. Completed pancreaticojejunal anastomosis. The anterior surface is overlapped with interrupted sutures of 3-0 silk. A short length of rubber catheter has been placed in the pancreatic duct to ensure its patency.

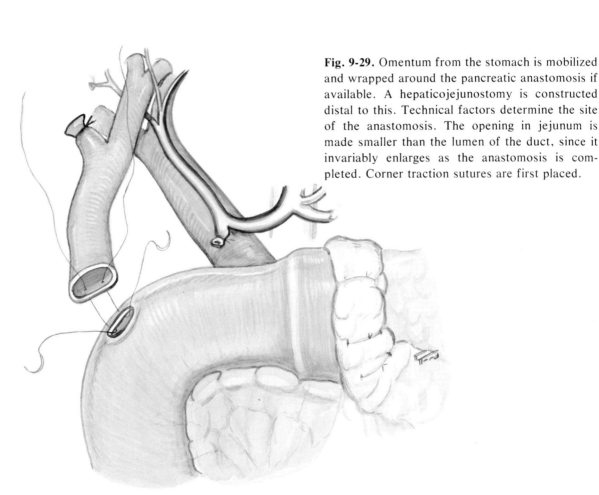

Fig. 9-29. Omentum from the stomach is mobilized and wrapped around the pancreatic anastomosis if available. A hepaticojejunostomy is constructed distal to this. Technical factors determine the site of the anastomosis. The opening in jejunum is made smaller than the lumen of the duct, since it invariably enlarges as the anastomosis is completed. Corner traction sutures are first placed.

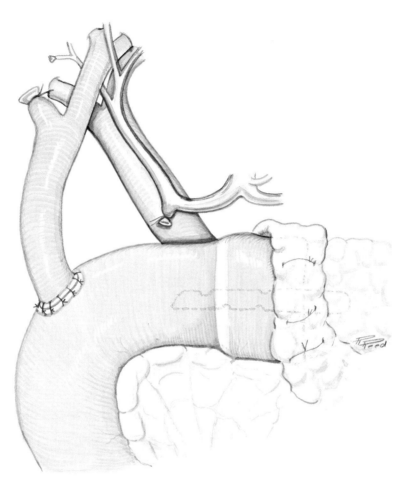

Fig. 9-30. The hepatojejunal anastomosis is completed in one or two layers. The inner layer (which approximates the mucosa) is made with absorbable 3-0 Dexon, and the outer layer with interrupted silk.

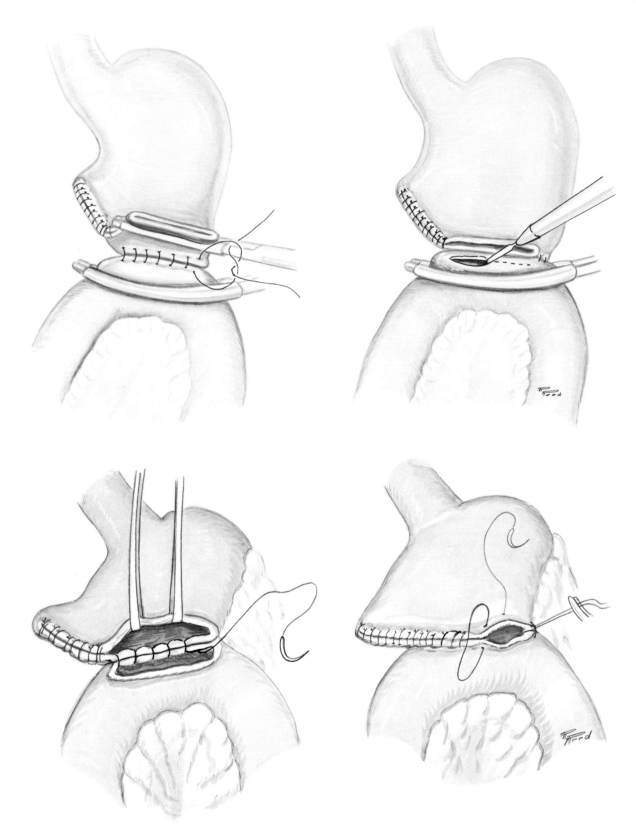

Fig. 9-31. An end-to-side gastrojejunostomy is made with an outer layer of 3-0 silk suture and an inner layer of continuous chromic catgut.

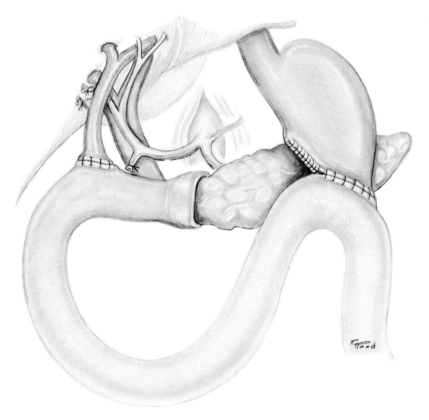

Fig. 9-32. Completed anastomosis. Sump drains have been placed around the pancreatico-jejunal union. (The omentum is removed for the purpose of illustration.)

Palliative surgery

Since most cancers of the head of the pancreas and periampullary area are unresectable, a palliative operation to relieve biliary and/or gastro-duodenal obstruction will be necessary for most patients. Although some authors have stated that survival is little improved by these operations, the argument is academic.[53] We believe that relief of jaundice and obstruction does improve the quality of the remaining time for most patients.

BILIARY ENTERIC BYPASS (Figs. 9-33 to 9-41)

There has been concern with what type of biliary intestinal bypass should be constructed for malignant biliary obstruction. Is a choledo-choenteric anastomosis preferred to a cholecystoenteric bypass? Is a Roux-en-Y or defunctionalized limb better than a loop anastomosis? Regardless of what method is used, there are two guiding principles to be followed: (1) decompress the liver and bile ducts and (2) place the bypass proximal to the obstruction.

Since survival with malignant obstruction is usually quite limited, from a practical standpoint any anastomosis conveniently and accurately constructed proximal to the obstructive point that will decompress the liver and biliary system is suitable.

Several studies have compared cholecystoenteric and choledochoenteric anastomoses. Experimental evidence has shown that in benign biliary obstruction there is less cholangitis and a greater fall in serum bilirubin after anastomosis of a defunctionalized limb of jejunum to the common bile duct than after a cholecystoenteric bypass. Richards and Sosin[56] noted little difference between these procedures in malignant diseases. Bufkin and co-workers[52] reported on 157 patients who underwent palliative surgery for malignant ductal obstruction: 83% of patients who had the gallbladder used for decompressive procedures were improved. When the two operations were compared for decline in serum bilirubin, a greater fall was noted after choledochojejunostomy than after cholecystoenteric bypass; but the common bile duct was employed in only five patients versus 141 in whom the gallbladder was used. Buckwalter and co-workers[51] reported a greater fall in serum bilirubin and slightly longer survival after choledochoenteric bypasses when compared to cholecystoenteric bypass.

We have no specific preference regarding which part of the biliary tree should be used to decompress the obstructed liver (assuming that both gallbladder and bile duct are suitable). The usual guiding principles have been emphasized. As a first step we perform cholangiography (using either gallbladder or common duct) to be certain that a long cystic duct paralleling the common duct is not present. If the cystic duct enters the common duct proximal to the obstruction, a cholecystoenteric bypass is made using either jejunum or duodenum. Most often a simple loop chole-cystojejunostomy (without an enteroanastomosis) is made. If cholelithiasis is present in an otherwise suitable gallbladder (not contracted or fibrotic), the stones may be removed prior to the construction of the anastomosis.

When carcinoma of the periampullary area is not resectable and obstructive jaundice is present, a biliary enteric bypass should be done to relieve the jaundice.

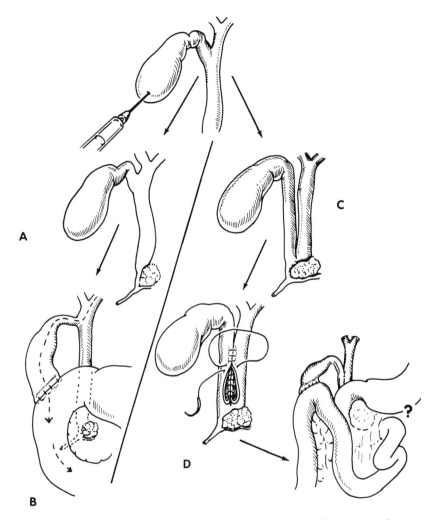

Fig. 9-33. A cholecystocholangiogram is first obtained to identify the site of entry of the cystic duct into the common duct. If the entry is well above the obstruction (**A**), a chole-cystoduodenostomy or cholecystojejunostomy can be made (**B**). At times a low entry of the cystic duct into the common duct is encountered (**C**). Then one of two alternatives is possible. Either (**C**) a choledochojejunostomy can be made proximal to the obstruction (and the gallbladder drained) or (**D**) the common duct can be anastomosed to the cystic duct and a cholecystoenteric anastomosis made. A gastrojejunostomy may or may not be done, depending on whether there is actual or impending gastric or duodenal obstruction.

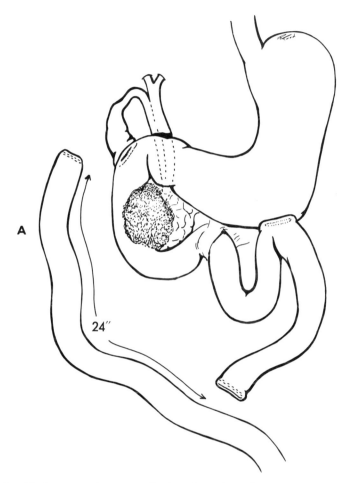

Fig. 9-34. A, In this instance, because of a low insertion of the cystic duct, a cholecysto-duodenostomy does not decompress the liver. Either the cystic duct can be joined to the common duct and the gallbladder used to decompress the hepatobiliary tree or a Roux-en-Y jejunal limb can be incorporated in a choledochojejunostomy.

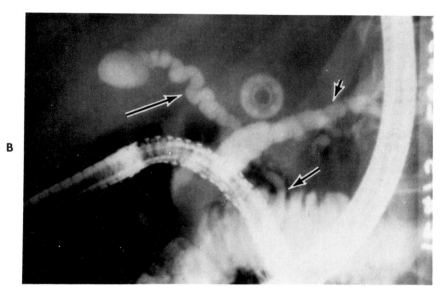

Fig. 9-34, cont'd. B, Endoscopic retrograde cholangiopancreatogram showing a dilated pancreatic duct (arrowhead) and a separate opening of the cystic duct into the duodenum (arrows). The obstructed common bile duct is not visualized. An unresectable pancreatic cancer was found at surgical exploration. In this instance a cholecystojejunostomy will not decompress the hepatobiliary tree. (Courtesy James Zelch, M.D., Hillcrest Hospital, Cleveland.)

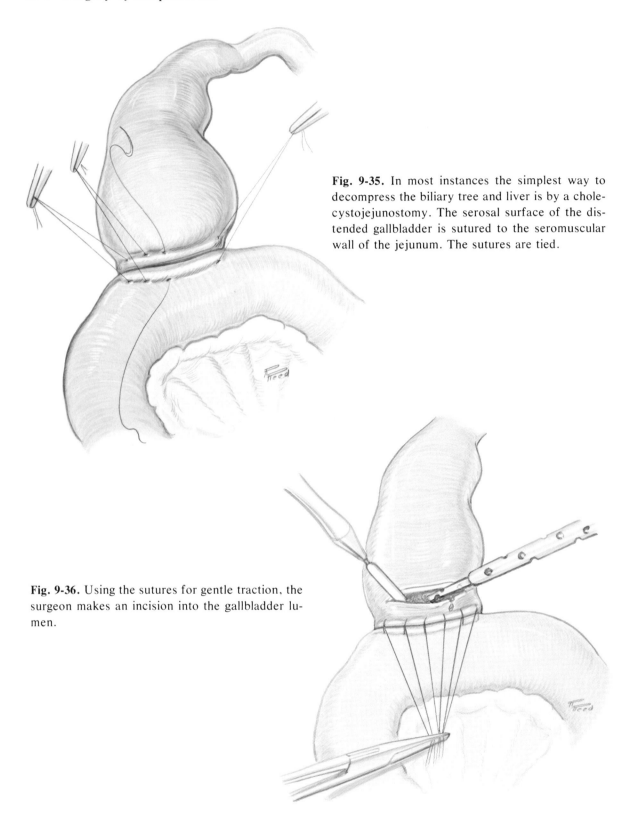

Fig. 9-35. In most instances the simplest way to decompress the biliary tree and liver is by a cholecystojejunostomy. The serosal surface of the distended gallbladder is sutured to the seromuscular wall of the jejunum. The sutures are tied.

Fig. 9-36. Using the sutures for gentle traction, the surgeon makes an incision into the gallbladder lumen.

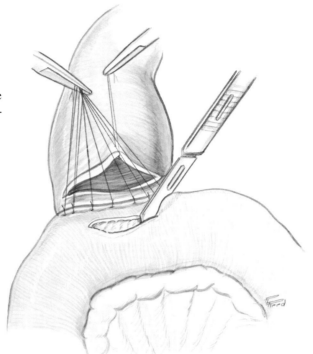

Fig. 9-37. A traction suture may be placed in the anterior wall of the gallbladder to facilitate suturing. A seromuscular jejunal incision is begun.

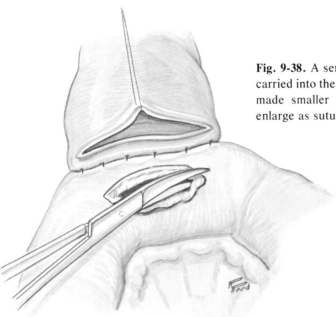

Fig. 9-38. A seromuscular incision is made and the incision carried into the lumen of the jejunum. The jejunal opening is made smaller than the gallbladder incision, since it will enlarge as sutures are placed.

Fig. 9-39. An inner layer of chromic catgut is then placed and tied. An anterior and posterior row of either continuous or interrupted sutures is continued to both corners.

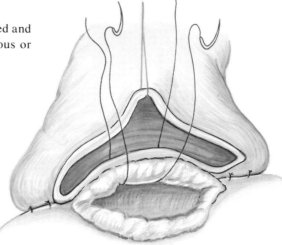

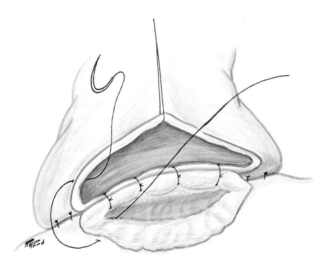

Fig. 9-40. The outer layer of interrupted nonabsorbable suture is placed and tied. If any signs of duodenal obstruction are present, an anterior gastrojejunostomy is made. The anastomosis is antecolic, side to side, and preferably near the pylorus.

Fig. 9-41. Completed operation.

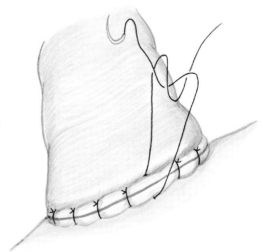

GASTRODUODENAL OBSTRUCTION

Up to 20% of patients with carcinoma of the pancreas have or will develop gastroduodenal obstruction (demonstrated by roentgen examinations or at surgery). In patients with symptomatic or imminent obstruction, there is no question about the need for a gastrojejunostomy. In patients with small pancreatic tumors that do not obstruct the stomach or duodenum, the decision to do a gastrojejunostomy may be more difficult.

Glassman and Johnston[55] noted that three of twenty patients required a secondary operation for gastric obstruction. Glantz and Ozeran[54] noted that five of twenty-two patients who had a biliary enteric bypass required additional surgery for gastric outlet obstruction. Richards and co-workers[56] noted that nineteen of fifty-six patients (34%) who survived biliary decompression and developed late gastric obstruction required operation. The obstruction appeared an average of 7 months after the first operation. Since survival is unpredictable with these neoplasms, it is difficult to predict in which patients delayed obstruction will develop.

We have no firm data or convictions about this issue. We have used gastroenteric bypass when gastric outlet obstruction is imminent or obvious at surgery. When small tumors are present and obstruction does not exist, we have elected not to do a gastroenteric bypass, taking the 10% chance of a reoperation if subsequent obstruction develops. Obviously this is a judgment decision: if there is any question of obstruction, we advise gastroenteric bypass.

DATA ON PALLIATIVE PROCEDURES

Personal statistics (S.O.H.) support our policy. A gastrojejunostomy need not be performed routinely at the time of a biliary bypass for obstructive jaundice—rather only if there is existing or impending duodenal obstruction. In an experience with 125 patients with carcinoma of the head of the pancreas, a simple biliary enteric bypass was carried out in eighty two patients and an accompanying anterior gastrojejunostomy in an additional ten patients (10/92, or about 10%). In only two patients was a later anterior gastrojejunostomy necessary, and in one it was done at a planned second-stage procedure.

Conservative approach

GEORGE CRILE, Jr.

In 1970 I reviewed the Cleveland Clinic's experience with the treatment of cancer of the pancreas and drew the following conclusion:

> Although some of the unusual types of pancreatic carcinomas and some of the small ones of the ducts may be cured by a radical operation, the average patient with an adenocarcinoma of the head of the pancreas that is big enough to be palpated will live longer and more comfortably if no attempt is made to take a biopsy specimen or to remove it. When nothing but adenocarcinoma of the head of the pancreas and only those large enough to be readily palpable are considered, radical operations appear to disseminate the disease and shorten life.[61]

At the time of that report, the Cleveland Clinic had no ten-year survivors of pancreaticoduodenectomy for adenocarcinoma of the head of the pancreas, and there still are none.

Since 1970 optimistic reports have continued to appear in which a significant number of cures of pancreatic carcinoma are described. With few exceptions, these reports fail to differentiate between the usual adenocarcinoma of the head of the pancreas and islet cell tumors, cystadenocarcinoma, and other rare and relatively benign tumors in the region. The most striking exception is reports from the Mayo Clinic which, in contrast to the experience of the rest of the world, continue to relate a relatively high proportion of long-term survivors after radical operations for the common type of adenocarcinoma of the pancreas.

Many authors report a much longer survival after the Whipple type of operation than after bypass, but invariably they fail to take into account two factors. One is the operative mortality, which is often as high as 50% and averages 32.1% according to the Commission on Professional and Hospital Activities (CPHA).[12a] If the patients who die from the operation are not included and only the survivors are counted, the reported average survival is a third longer than the true average. The second factor is that the patients who are selected for the radical operation are, by definition, in a more favorable stage of the disease or in better general condition than those who are treated palliatively by a bypass procedure. Naturally the healthier patients who survive the radical operation live longer than the poor-risk patients, who are treated conservatively. This would be true even if the radical operation did no good at all or did only a little harm.

Shapiro[83] collected the results of seventeen series of pancreaticoduodenectomy (496 cases) and found that the operative mortality rate was 21% and the five-year survivors 4%. Some of these patients may have had tumors other than the ordinary adenocarcinoma, and some may have died of cancer after the five-year period. Moreover, the mortality rates and survival rates in *reported* series usually are better than in cases which remain unreported. In confirmation of this the CPHA, checking on 271 radical pancreaticoduodenectomies done in the hospitals it audits, found the average mortality rate to be 10% higher than the 21% mortality in the published series.

In twenty articles 703 radical resections for cancer of the pancreas were reported. If the Mayo Clinic results[76] (so different from all the others) are excluded, ten of 703 patients appear to have been cured—1.4% of those subjected to the radical operation. Several lived five years and were excluded as cures because they later died of cancer, and several were excluded because the cancer was islet cell or cystadenocarcinoma. In four of the six reports in which there were five-year survivors, it is impossible to tell what type of cancer was treated or whether there were recurrences after five years. The actual cure rate of patients subjected to pancreaticoduodenectomy for ordinary adenocarcinoma of the pancreas, excluding the Mayo Clinic series, cannot therefore exceed 1%. The price for this 1% salvage is a mortality rate that in the reported series averages 26% and throughout the United States averages 32.1% (CPHA).

Most patients with cancer of the pancreas are in their 60s or 70s; thus even if they are cured by a radical operation, their life expectancy is not likely to be more than ten years. The average survival of a good-risk patient with localized disease who is treated by a bypass instead of by a radical pancreaticoduodenectomy is 12 months. When the patient dies postoperatively as a result of a radical operation, approximately a year of life which would have resulted from a bypass is sacrificed. On the average, the survivor of the radical operation has a life expectancy of ten years. Against these ten years gained, twenty-six years of life expectancy have been lost as a result of the deaths of twenty-six of the 100 patients treated by the radical operation, almost all of whom would have survived a bypass. The total number of patient–years of life lost by trying to effect a cure is at least ten.

It is thus clear that a surgeon's mortality rate for the radical operation must be under 10% if he is to come out ahead with the big operation. Moreover, patients with proved cancer have survived five years and more after bypass alone—a large part of the life expectancy of people in their late 60s and 70s. Ficarra[63] reported that two patients who survived more than five years proved at autopsy to have had cancer; and two of the Massachusetts General patients treated by bypass instead of resection lived for five years. If more of the favorable cancers which are treated routinely by resection were treated by bypass, it is likely that a higher proportion of the patients would live five years. Despite most authors' conclusions, therefore, the evidence does not support the routine use of pancreaticoduodenectomy for operable adenocarcinoma of the pancreas.

Aggressive approach

JOHN W. BRAASCH

This chapter, on the indications for and technique of the Whipple operation for neoplastic disease, assumes a moderate stance with regard to the procedure. In the final analysis, one's opinion concerning pancreaticoduodenectomy is influenced heavily by the local operative mortality for the operation. Thus with carcinoma of the pancreas (which has a low five-year survival after resection) there must be a low operative mortality to justify the operation. With careful attention to the pancreaticojejunostomy, with avoidance of the high-risk situations of deep jaundice and infection, and with the change to total pancreatectomy when the pancreas and duct are unfavorable for anastomosis, I believe a less than 10% mortality is achievable. It is therefore desirable to use this operation for carcinoma of the pancreatic head in favorable circumstances (e.g., with negative nodes).

Islet cell tumors of the head of the pancreas are best treated by excision of the tumor with a small rim of pancreatic tissue. The incidence of malignancy in an islet cell tumor without obvious metastases is less than the operative mortality of the Whipple procedure even in the most experienced hands.

The authors have mentioned the chance for error in identifying the primary site of periampullary carcinoma. Thus 10% to 20% of tumors thought to arise in the head of the pancreas actually are primary in the distal bile duct. With the relatively favorable outlook for resected lower bile duct tumors, lesions of the head possibly arising in the lower duct should be resected.

I agree that malignancies clearly of the duodenum, ampulla, and lower bile duct need resection; however, I would resect them even with positive first-echelon nodes (common duct and gastroduodenal nodes). Again a pancreas unfavorable for anastomosis should be totally removed.

Of great importance technically is the placement of drains suitable for preventing the accumulation of activated pancreatic enzymes in the retroperitoneal area. To this end, four sump drains and two Penrose drains are positioned behind the anastomoses. These are suitable for irrigation and drainage. Should an obvious leak appear from the pancreatic or biliary tract anastomosis, Ringer's lactate solution may be introduced in a constant infusion through two of the sump drains and suction applied to the other two. Thus the vulnerable area of the gastroduodenal artery stump and the inferior vena cava is continually bathed in Ringer's lactate solution, which carries away with it the activated pancreatic enzymes.

The Cleveland Clinic has done a valuable service to surgery in calling attention to the dangers of pancreaticoduodenectomy and to the fact that the operating surgeon must weigh these dangers against the possible benefits of the procedure, which are marginal in carcinoma of the pancreas.

REFERENCES
Periampullary carcinoma

1. Aston, S. J., and Longmire, W. P., Jr.: Pancreaticoduodenal resection: twenty years experience, Arch. Surg. **106**:813, 1973.

2. Baylor, S. M., and Berg, J. W.: Cross-classification and survival characteristics of 5,000 cases of cancer of the pancreas, J. Surg. Oncol. **5**:335, 1973.

2a. Berman, L. G., Prior, J. T., Abramow, S. M., and Ziegler, D. D.: A study of the pancreatic duct in man by the use of vinyl acetate casts of postmortem preparations, Surg. Gynecol. Obstet. **110**:391, 1960.

3. Beall, M. S., Dyer, G. A., and Stephenson, H.E., Jr.: Disappointments in the management of patients with malignancy of pancreas, duodenum, and common bile duct, Arch. Surg. **101**:461, 1970.

4. Braasch, J. W., and Camer, S. J.: Periampullary carcinoma, Med. Clin. N. Am. **59**:309, 1975.

5. Braasch, J. W., Warren, K. W., and Kune, G. A.: Malignant neoplasms of the bile ducts, Surg. Clin. North Am. **47**:627, 1967.

6. Bruno, M. S., and Fein, H. D.: Primary malignant and benign tumors of the duodenum: a study of 18 cases stressing the clinical and roentgenographic features, Arch. Intern. Med. **125**:670, 1970.

7. Brunschwig, A.: Resection of the head of the pancreas and duodenum for carcinoma—pancreaticoduodenectomy, Surg. Gynecol. Obstet. **65**:681, 1937.

8. Buckwalter, J. A., Lawton, R. L., and Tidrick, R. T.: Pancreatoduodenectomy, Arch. Surg. **89**:331, 1964.

9. Bufkin, W. J., Smith, P. E., and Krementz, E. T.: Evaluation of palliative operations for carcinoma of the pancreas, Arch. Surg. **94**:240, 1967.

10. Burgerman, A., Baggenstoss, A. H., and Cain, J. C.: Primary malignant neoplasms of the duodenum, excluding the papilla of Vater; clinicopathologic study of 31 cases, Gastroenterology **30**:421, 1956.

11. Child, C. G., III, Holswade, G. R., McClure, R. D., Jr., Gore, A. L., and O'Neill, E. A.: Pancreaticoduodenectomy with resection of portal vein in the Macaca mulatta monkey and in man, Surg. Gynecol. Obstet. **94**:31, 1952.

12. Clouse, M. E., Gregg, J. A., and Sedgwick, C. E.: Angiography vs. pancreatography in the diagnosis of carcinoma of the pancreas, Radiology **114**:605, 1975.

12a. Commission on Professional and Hospital Activities (CPHA): Cancer Registry Information System, Ann Arbor, Mich., 1975.

13. Cooperman, A. M., Warner, D., Hoerr, S. O., Hermann R. E., and Esselstyn, C. B., Jr.: Cancer of the duodenum. (In preparation.)

14. Crile, G., Jr.: The advantages of bypass operations over radical pancreatoduodenectomy in the treatment of pancreatic carcinoma, Surg. Gynecol. Obstet. **130**:1049, 1970.

15. Elias, E., Hamlyn, A. N., Jain, S., Long, R. G., Summerfield, J. A., Dick, R., and Sherlock, S.: A randomized trial of percutaneous transhepatic cholangiography with the Chiba needle versus the endoscopic retrograde cholangiography for bile duct visualization in jaundice, Gastroenterology **71**:439, 1976.

16. Feduska, N. J., Dent, T. L., and Lindenauer, S. M.: Results of palliative operations for carcinoma of the pancreas, Arch. Surg. **103**:330, 1971.

17. Fortner, J. G.: Regional resection of cancer of the pancreas: a new surgical approach, Surgery **73**:307, 1973.

18. Gatti, D. J., O'Brien, P. H. and Grooms, G. A.: Analysis of pancreaticoduodenectomy, South. Med. J. **67**:278, 1974.

19. Glenn, F., and Thorbjarnarson, B.: Carcinoma of the pancreas, Ann. Surg. **159**:945, 1964.

20. Gray, L. W., Jr., Crook, J. N., and Cohn, I., Jr.: Carcinoma of the pancreas, Proc. Natl. Cancer Conf. **7:**503, 1973.

21. Halsted, W. S.: Contributions to the surgery of the bile passages, especially of the common bile duct, Boston Med. Surg. J. **141:**645, 1899.

22. Hermreck, A. S., Thomas, C. Y., IV, and Friesen, S. R.: Importance of pathologic staging in the surgical management of adenocarcinoma of the exocrine pancreas, Am. J. Surg. **127:**653, 1974.

23. Hicks, R. E., and Brooks, J. R.: Total pancreatectomy for ductal carcinoma, Surg. Gynecol. Obstet. **133:**16, 1971.

24. Hoffman, R. E., and Donegan, W. L.: Experience with pancreatoduodenectomy in a cancer hospital, Am. J. Surg. **129:**292, 1975.

24a. Hollinshead, H.: Anatomy for surgeons. Vol. 2. The thorax, abdomen, and pelvis, New York, 1956, Harper & Bros.

25. Hubbard, T. B., Jr.: Carcinoma of the head of the pancreas: resection of the portal vein and portocaval shunt, Ann. Surg. **147:**935, 1958.

26. Hunt, V. C.: Surgical management of carcinoma of the ampulla of Vater and of the periampullary portion of the duodenum, Ann. Surg. **114:**570, 1941.

27. Jefferson, G.: Carcinoma of the supra-papillary duodenum casually associated with pre-existing simple ulcer, Br. J. Surg. **4:**209, 1916.

28. Kenefick, J. S.: Carcinoma of the duodenum, Br. J. Surg. **59:**50, 1972.

29. Lansing, P. B., Blalock, J. B., and Ochsner, J. L.: Pancreatoduodenectomy. A respective review 1949-1969, Am. Surgeon **38:**79, 1972.

30. Lund, F.: Carcinoma of the pancreas: palliative or radical surgery? Acta Chir. Scand. **134:**461, 1968.

30a. Mackie, J. A., Rhoads, J. E., and Park, C. D.: Pancreaticogastrostomy: a further evaluation, Ann. Surg. **181:**541, 1975.

31. Makipour, H., Cooperman, A. M., Danzi, J. T., and Farmer, R. G.: Carcinoma of the ampulla of Vater; review of 38 cases with emphasis on treatment and prognostic factors, Ann. Surg. **183:**341, 1976.

32. McDermott, W. V., Jr.: One stage pancreaticoduodenectomy with resection of the portal vein for carcinoma of the pancreas, Ann. Surg. **136:**1012, 1952.

33. Mongé, J. J.: Survival of patients with small carcinomas of the head of the pancreas, Ann. Surg. **166:**908, 1967.

34. Mongé, J. J., Dockerty, M. B., Wollaeger, E. E., and Malcolm, B.: Clinico-pathologic observations on radical pancreatoduodenal resection for peripapillary carcinoma, Surg. Gynecol. Obstet. **118:**275, 1964.

35. Mongé, J. J., Judd, E. S., and Gage, R. P.: Radical pancreaticoduodenectomy; a 22-year experience with the complications, mortality rate and survival rate, Ann. Surg. **160:**711, 1964.

36. Morris, J. P., and Nardi, G. L.: Pancreaticoduodenal cancer. Experience from 1951 to 1960 with a look ahead and behind, Arch. Surg. **92:**834, 1966.

37. Nakase, A., Matsumoto, Y., Uchida, K., and Honjo, I.: Surgical treatment of cancer of the pancreas and the periampullary region: cumulative results in 57 institutions in Japan, Ann. Surg. **185:**52, 1977.

37a. Pliam, M. B., and ReMine, W. H.: Further evaluation of total pancreatectomy, Arch. Surg. **110:**506, 1975.

38. Pope, N. A., and Fish, J. C.: Palliative surgery for carcinoma of the pancreas, Am. J. Surg. **121:**271, 1971.

39. Ross, D. E.: Cancer of the pancreas, a plea for total pancreatectomy, Am. J. Surg. **87:**20, 1954.

40. Shapiro, T. M.: Adenocarcinoma of the pancreas: a statistical analysis of biliary

bypass vs. Whipple resection in good-risk patients, Ann. Surg. **182:**715, 1975.

41. van Heerden, J. A., Judd, F. S., and Dockerty, M. B.: Carcinoma of the extrahepatic bile ducts. A clinicopathologic study, Am. J. Surg. **113:**49, 1967.
42. Warren, K. W. Cited by Pope, N. A., and Fish, J. C.: Am. J. Surg. **121:**271, 1971.
43. Warren, K. W.: Current concepts in management of periampullary carcinoma, Am. Surg. **39:**667, 1973.
44. Warren, K. W., Braasch, J. W., and Thum, C. W.: Diagnosis and surgical treatment of carcinoma of the pancreas, Curr. Probl. Surg. p. 3, June, 1968.
45. Warren, K. W., Choe, D. S., Plaza, J., and Relihan, M.: Results of radical resection for periampullary cancer, Ann. Surg. **181:**534, 1975.
46. Whipple, A. O.: The rationale of radical surgery for cancer of the pancreas and ampullary region, Ann. Surg. **114:**612, 1941.
47. Whipple, A. O.: Pancreaticoduodenectomy for islet cell carcinoma: a five-year follow-up, Surgery **121:**847, 1945.
48. Whipple, A. O., Parsons, W. B., and Mullins, C. R.: Treatment of carcinoma of ampulla of Vater, Ann. Surg. **102:**763, 1935.
49. Wilson, S. M., and Block, G. E.: Periampullary carcinoma, Arch. Surg. **108:**539, 1974.
50. Wise, L., Pizzimbono, C., and Denner, L.: Periampullary cancer: a clinicopathological study of 62 patients, Am. J. Surg. **131:**141, 1976.

Palliative surgery

51. Buckwalter, J. A., Lawton, R. L., and Tidrick, R. T.: Bypass operations for neoplastic biliary tract obstruction, Am. J. Surg. **109:**100, 1965.
52. Bufkin, W. J., Prentiss, E., Smith, M. D., and Krementz, E. T.: Evaluation of palliative operations for carcinoma of the pancreas, Arch. Surg. **94:**240, 1967.
53. Feduska, N. J., Dent, T. L., and Lindenauer, S. M.: Results of palliative operations for carcinoma of the pancreas, Arch. Surg. **103:**330, 1971.
54. Glantz, G., and Ozeran, R. S.: Role of gastroenterostomy in management of pancreatic carcinoma: risk of duodenal obstruction after biliary bypass, Am. Surg. **32:**670, 1966.
55. Glassman, W. S., and Johnston, P. W.: Palliative surgery in carcinoma of the pancreas, Geriatrics **10:**456, 1955.
56. Richards, A. B., and Sosin, H.: Cancer of the pancreas: the value of radical and palliative surgery, Ann. Surg. **177:**325, 1973.

Conservative approach

57. Aston, S. J., and Longmire, W. P., Jr.: Pancreaticoduodenal resection, Arch. Surg. **106:**813, 1973.
58. Beall, M. S., Dyer, G. A., and Stephenson, H. E., Jr.: Disappointments in the management of patients with malignancy of pancreas, duodenum, and common bile duct, Arch. Surg. **101:**461, 1970.
59. Bowden, L., and Pack, G. T.: Cancer of the pancreas. A collective review of the experiences of the gastric service of the Memorial Cancer Center, 1926-1958, GEN **23:**339, 1969.
60. Buckwalter, J. A., Lawton, R. L., and Tidrick, R. T.: Pancreatoduodenectomy, Arch. Surg. **89:**331, 1964.
61. Crile, G., Jr.: The advantages of bypass operations over radical pancreatoduodenectomy in the treatment of pancreatic carcinoma, Surg. Gynecol. Obstet. **130:**1049, 1970.
62. Feduska, N. J., Dent, T. L., and Lindenauer, S. M.: Results of palliative operations for carcinoma of the pancreas, Arch. Surg. **103:**330, 1971.
63. Ficarra, B. J.: Conservative surgery for pancreatic cancer in geriatric patients, J. Am. Geriatr. Soc. **20:**560, 1972.

64. Fish, J. C., and Cleveland, B. A.: Pancreaticoduodenectomy for peri-ampullary carcinoma, Ann. Surg. **159**:469, 1964.
65. Glenn, F., and Thorbjarnarson, B.: Carcinoma of the pancreas, Ann. Surg. **159**:945, 1964.
66. Hermreck, A. S., Thomas, C. Y., IV, and Friesen, S. R.: Importance of pathologic staging in the surgical management of adenocarcinoma of the exocrine pancreas, Am. J. Surg. **127**:653, 1974.
67. Hertzberg, J.: Pancreatico-duodenal resection and bypass operation in patients with carcinoma of the head of the pancreas, ampulla, and distal end of the common duct, Acta Chir. Scand. **140**:523, 1973.
68. Hoffman, R. D.: Experience with pancreatoduodenectomy in a cancer hospital, Am. J. Surg. **129**:292, 1975.
69. Jordan, G. L., Jr.: Surgical management of carcinoma of the pancreas and peri-ampullary region, Am. J. Surg. **107**:313, 1964.
70. Judd, E. S.: Discussion in Mongé, J. J., Judd, E. S., and Gage, R. P.: Ann. Surg. **160**:711, 1964.
71. Koivuniemi, M. L., Lempinen, M., and Pantzar, P.: Fine-needle aspiration biopsy of pancreas, Ann. Chir. Gynaecol. Fenn. **61**:273, 1972.
72. Lansing, P. B., Blalock, P. B., and Ochsner, J. L.: Pancreaticoduodenectomy: a retrospective review, 1949-1969, Am. Surg. **38**:79, 1972.
73. Lightwood, R.: Surgical Congress News, vol. 4, no. 5, May, 1976.
74. Lund, F.: Carcinoma of the pancreas, Acta Chir. Scand. **134**:461, 1968.
75. McDermott, W. V., Jr.: Discussion in Mongé, J. J., Judd, E. S., and Gage, R. P.: Ann. Surg. **160**:711, 1964.
76. Mongé, J. J., Judd, E. S., and Gage, R. P..: Radial pancreaticoduodenectomy; a 22-year experience with the complications, mortality rate, and survival rate, Ann. Surg. **160**:711, 1964.
77. Morris, P. J.: Pancreaticoduodenal cancer, Arch. Surg. **92**:834, 1966.
78. Najera, E., and White, R.: Carcinoma of the pancreas, Arch. Surg. **106**:293, 1973.
79. Porter, M. R.: Carcinoma of the pancreaticoduodenal area, Ann. Surg. **148**:711, 1958.
80. Ruilova, L. A., and Hershey, G. B.: Experience with 21 pancreaticoduodenectomies, Arch. Surg. **111**:27, 1976.
81. Salmon, P. A.: Carcinoma of the pancreas and extrahepatic biliary system, Surgery **60**:554, 1966.
82. Schultz, N. J., and Sanders, R. J.: Evaluation of pancreatic biopsy, Ann. Surg. **158**:1053, 1963.
83. Shapiro, T. M.: Adenocarcinoma of the pancreas: a statistical analysis of biliary bypass vs. Whipple resection in good-risk patients, Ann. Surg. **182**:715, 1975.
84. Smith, P. E.: An analysis of 600 patients with carcinoma of the pancreas, Surg. Gynecol. Obstet. **124**:1288, 1967.
85. Tepper, J., Nardi, G., and Suit, H.: Carcinoma of the pancreas: review of MGH experience from 1963 to 1973, Cancer **37**:1519, 1976.
86. Warren, K. W., Cattell, R. B., Blackburn, J. P., and Nora, P. F.: A long-term appraisal of pancreaticoduodenal resection for peri-ampullary carcinoma, Ann. Surg. **155**:652, 1962.
87. White, T. T.: Surgical anatomy of the pancreas. In Carey, L. C., editor: The pancreas, St. Louis, 1973, The C. V. Mosby Co.
88. Womack, N. Discussion in Brunschweig, A.: Pancreatoduodenectomy, Ann. Surg. **136**:610, 1952.

CHAPTER 10

Endocrine diseases of the pancreas

Insulinomas

ROBERT E. HERMANN

HISTORICAL PROFILE

1902   Islet cell tumor of pancreas identified as an adenoma (Nicholls[5])

1922   Discovery of insulin by Banting, Best, and Macleod

1924   Correlation between islet cell adenomas and hyperinsulinism proposed (Harris[4])

1927   Islet cell carcinoma with metastases found at operation in a patient with hyperinsulinism (Wilder et al.[7])

1929   Islet cell adenoma removed, with relief of hypoglycemic symptoms (Campbell et al.[2])

1935   "Whipple's triad" established (Whipple and Frantz[6])

THE LESION

The beta cells of the islets of Langerhans secrete insulin. These cells are hyperactive in insulinomas. Microscopically they tend to group in alveolar formation or even ductlike structures. To diagnose malignancy, the pathologist may have to depend on features other than the microscopic appearance and organization: size (larger than 3 cm), invasion of adjacent structures, presence of metastases, perineural invasion.

Grossly, benign insulinomas tend to be well localized with a loose areolar capsule, more reddish brown and firmer than the yellowish and relatively soft pancreatic acinar tissue. They are solitary tumors and benign in 90% of the reported cases. In about 10% of the cases, the adenomas are multiple; and there have been sporadic reports of beta cell hyperplasia or multiple adenomatosis. About 90% can be visualized or palpated at operation, but some 10% are occult and defy identification after the most careful and thorough exploration. Roughly one third of the tumors lie in the head and uncinate process of the pancreas. One third are in the body. One third are in the tail. (This fact supports "blind" resection of the body and tail if a lesion cannot be identified since the odds are two out of three that the tumor will be included in the removed tissues.) An occasional adenoma will be found in any location where aberrant pancreatic tissue may occur, most commonly in the wall of the abdomen.

DIAGNOSIS

The onset of symptoms resulting from overproduction of insulin by beta cell tumors may be insidious. The symptoms vary from subtle feelings of nervousness, tremulousness, weakness, and lethargy to obvious personality changes or attacks of syncope. *Whipple's triad* has been and remains the most important basis for a clinical diagnosis of insulinoma:

1. Symptoms of hypoglycemia brought on by fasting
2. Serum glucose levels below 50 mg/dl
3. Relief of all symptoms by the administration of glucose.

Nevertheless, the diagnosis is not always an easy one; functional and factitial hypoglycemia as well as the hypoglycemia produced by rare large mesenchymal neoplasms must be ruled out. Occasionally, symptomatic hypoglycemia is actually a rebound phenomenon in diabetes mellitus.

A careful diagnostic workup is essential for the welfare of the patient and for the peace of mind of the surgeon, who may experience difficulty in locating the lesion at operation. Confidence in the accuracy of the preoperative diagnosis is essential if the surgeon is to perform correctly in this dilemma. A prolonged fast is still a mainstay of clinical diagnosis, but serum insulin levels and C-peptide analysis are newer and less imposing tests that are helpful in establishing the diagnosis. At the Cleveland Clinic we have found selective celiac and superior mesenteric arteriography to be beneficial, though not infallible, in roentgenographically localizing these lesions and lending strong support to the positive diagnosis of insulinoma.

Surgical technique

Once the diagnosis of organic hypoglycemia has been made and an arteriogram (Fig. 10-1) confirming the presence or indicating the location of an adenoma obtained, the optimal treatment for this problem is surgical excision of the insulinoma.

The surgeon widely exposes the pancreas by dividing the gastrocolic omentum and elevating the stomach (Fig. 10-2). He then performs a wide Kocher maneuver so the head and uncinate process of the gland can be bimanually palpated (Fig. 10-3). In addition, he can elevate the body and tail by incising along the lower border of the gland and bimanually palpating the distal half of the pancreas (Fig. 10-4). Attention should be directed initially to any suspicious area. In addition, the surgeon should carefully palpate the antrum of the stomach and the entire duodenum and should look for a Meckel's diverticulum, because ectopic pancreatic tissue may rarely be found in these locations.

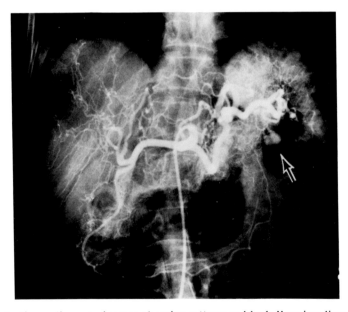

Fig. 10-1. Selective celiac arteriogram showing a "tumor blush," an insulinoma (arrow) in the tail of the pancreas.

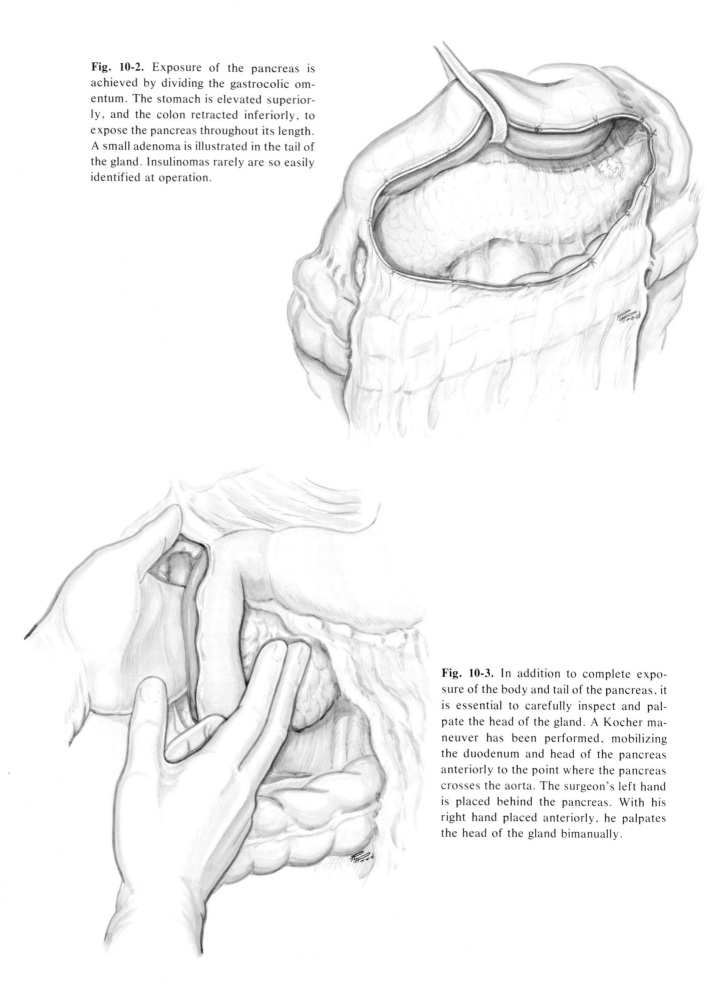

Fig. 10-2. Exposure of the pancreas is achieved by dividing the gastrocolic omentum. The stomach is elevated superiorly, and the colon retracted inferiorly, to expose the pancreas throughout its length. A small adenoma is illustrated in the tail of the gland. Insulinomas rarely are so easily identified at operation.

Fig. 10-3. In addition to complete exposure of the body and tail of the pancreas, it is essential to carefully inspect and palpate the head of the gland. A Kocher maneuver has been performed, mobilizing the duodenum and head of the pancreas anteriorly to the point where the pancreas crosses the aorta. The surgeon's left hand is placed behind the pancreas. With his right hand placed anteriorly, he palpates the head of the gland bimanually.

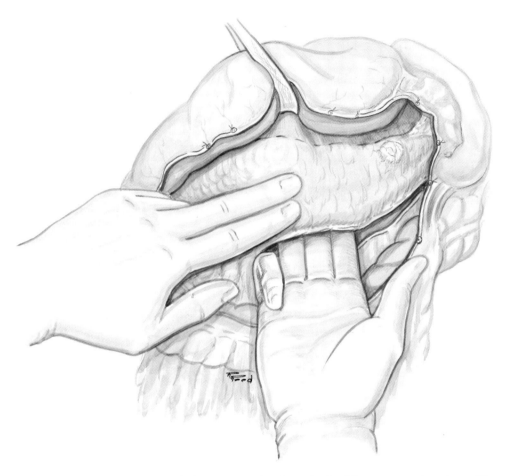

Fig. 10-4. The lower border of the pancreas has been incised in an avascular plane. The surgeon has passed his right hand up behind the gland, again to permit bimanual palpation of the body and tail of the pancreas. An islet cell tumor is located in the tail of the gland.

If the adenoma is palpated in the body or tail of the pancreas, a distal pancreatectomy removing the lesion usually is performed (Figs. 10-5 and 10-6). If the lesion is near the inferior border (away from the main pancreatic duct), it may be excised by wedge resection between hemoclips.

When a solitary adenoma is found in the head of the pancreas or the uncinate process, it is carefully enucleated (Figs. 10-7 to 10-11). Most insulinomas will separate easily from normal pancreas. Careful ligation of the blood vessels entering the adenoma can be performed with the use of fine silver clips. If an adenoma larger than 3 cm in the head of the pancreas is difficult to enucleate, is intensely vascular, or has any characteristics of malignancy identifiable to the pathologist after enucleation—then a Whipple resection of the entire head of the pancreas is performed. The presence of metastases, of course, will establish the malignant character of the primary growth.

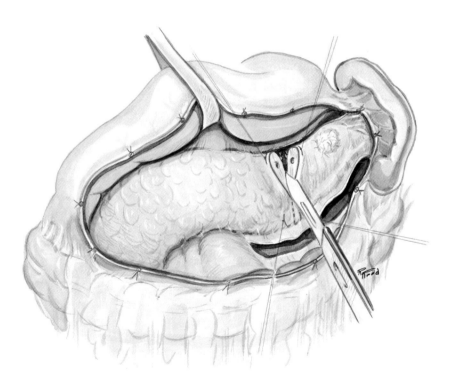

Fig. 10-5. Having identified an adenoma in the distal pancreas, the surgeon mobilizes the tail of the gland and the spleen anteriorly, dividing their retroperitoneal attachments. The splenic vessels are ligated separately on the posterior side of the pancreas, and the gland is divided. The tail, with the insulinoma, is removed. Traction sutures of 3-0 silk help stabilize or hold the gland. The spleen is removed with the tail of the pancreas.

It is to be emphasized that a Whipple procedure for all lesions found in the head of the pancreas is unwise. Ninety percent of insulinomas are benign, and most small lesions can be enucleated easily.

If for any reason the surgeon suspects that there are multiple adenomas in the pancreas or adenomatosis, then blood glucose levels are monitored intraoperatively. If multiple lesions are found, a subtotal pancreatectomy can be performed, removing 80% or 85% of the pancreas (Fig. 10-12).

If the insulinoma is an occult lesion (i.e., no tumor can be seen or palpated), we first resect an estimated two thirds of the pancreas—all the gland to the left of the superior mesenteric vessels. Blood glucose levels are monitored while the pathologist searches for a small adenoma in the resected tissue. If the blood glucose level does not rise within the next 30 or 40 minutes, it may be advisable to remove additional distal pancreas (Fig. 10-13). We do not do a total pancreatectomy at the intial operative procedure; rather we close the abdomen and assess the patient postoperatively for relief of symptoms.

The operative mortality for excision of insulinoma was reviewed by Filipi and Higgins[3] and found to be approximately 5% when enucleation of an adenoma or distal pancreatectomy was performed. With a subtotal

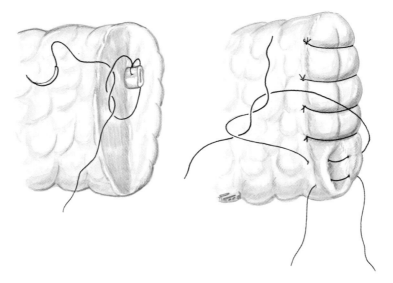

Fig. 10-6. After the pancreas has been divided, hemostasis of small vessels is achieved with silk ligatures or the electrocautery. The main pancreatic duct should be separately isolated and ligated, or it should be suture ligated with 3-0 silk as in this illustration. The divided gland is then oversewn with interrupted 3-0 silk sutures or mattress sutures to close the cut edge. This maneuver is facilitated by wedging the remaining stump toward the center of the gland. The divided pancreas should be drained with a Penrose or sump suction drain.

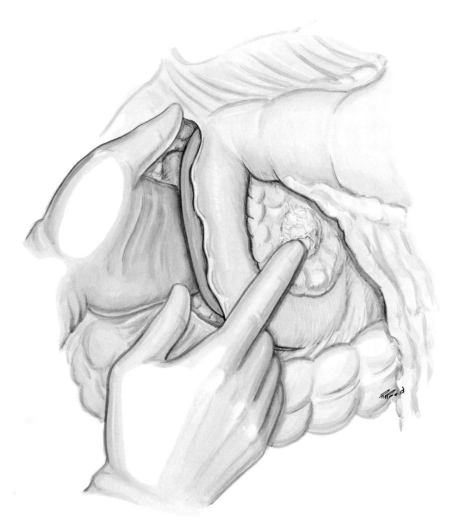

Fig. 10-7. The surgeon's right hand is palpating an islet cell adenoma in the head of the pancreas while his left hand offers resistance behind the gland, pushing the adenoma forward.

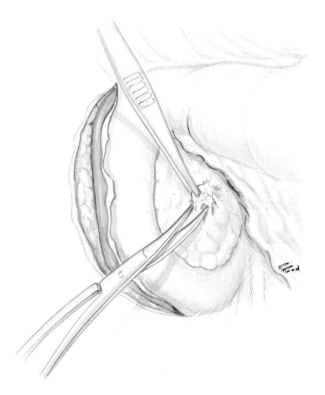

Fig. 10-8. The adenoma is grasped by a forceps and carefully removed from the surrounding normal gland by sharp and blunt dissection. Most adenomas separate fairly easily with an identifiable cleavage plane around them.

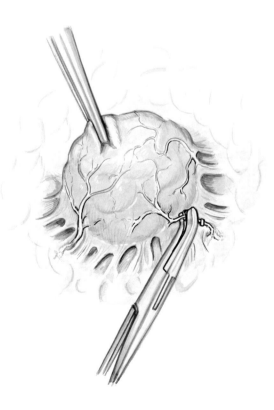

Fig. 10-9. Small blood vessels feeding the adenoma are individually ligated with fine "silver" clips. This is an excellent method of hemostasis as the adenoma is removed.

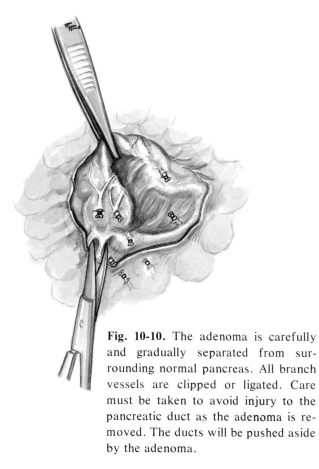

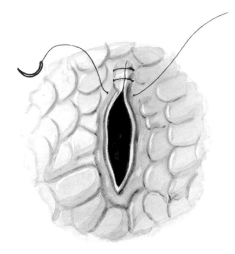

Fig. 10-10. The adenoma is carefully and gradually separated from surrounding normal pancreas. All branch vessels are clipped or ligated. Care must be taken to avoid injury to the pancreatic duct as the adenoma is removed. The ducts will be pushed aside by the adenoma.

Fig. 10-11. The defect in the capsule of the pancreas is closed with interrupted 3-0 silk sutures after enucleation of the adenoma. A drain or sump suction tube is placed in case there is some leakage of pancreatic juice postoperatively.

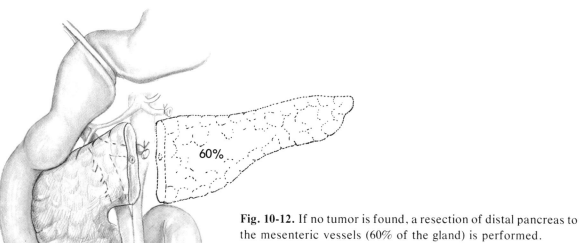

Fig. 10-12. If no tumor is found, a resection of distal pancreas to the mesenteric vessels (60% of the gland) is performed.

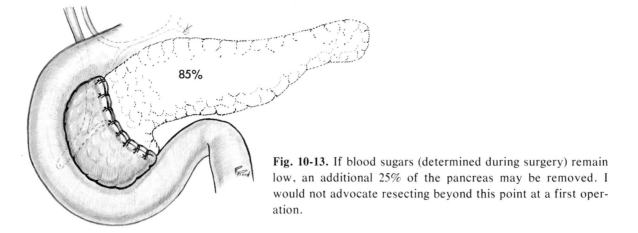

Fig. 10-13. If blood sugars (determined during surgery) remain low, an additional 25% of the pancreas may be removed. I would not advocate resecting beyond this point at a first operation.

pancreatectomy or a Whipple procedure the operative mortality was doubled.[3]

When a distal pancreatectomy has been performed, we oversew the remaining cut end carefully ligating the main pancreatic duct. Some surgeons routinely drain the divided distal pancreas by anastomosing it to a Roux-en-Y jejunal loop. We have not found this to be necessary when the gland is normal. Drains are always placed in the operative site near the resected edge of the pancreas and are brought out through a separate stab incision. When an adenoma has been enucleated from the head of the pancreas, the defect should be carefully repaired by interrupted 3-0 silk sutures. Great care must be taken to ligate or clip any small pancreatic ducts which may have been inadvertently divided. The site of enucleation should be drained through a separate stab wound.

POSTOPERATIVE COURSE

After surgery most patients experience a rebound hyperglycemia for 5 or 6 days. These elevated blood glucose levels gradually return to normal after the first postoperative week. We do not routinely administer insulin postoperatively, because this hyperglycemia is a stimulus for the remaining suppressed islet tissue to regain its normal function. Only if a subtotal pancreatectomy has been performed, with very little remaining pancreatic tissue, do we consider the use of insulin postoperatively.

The drains left in the region of the pancreas may gradually be removed after 4 or 5 days. Most patients are discharged from the hospital 7 to 10 days after operation. Occasionally, prolonged pancreatic leakage occurs with a temporary fistula. If there is no pancreatic duct obstruction, these pancreatic fistulas almost always close spontaneously in several weeks or, rarely, a month or longer.

Pancreatic cholera—the watery diarrhea syndrome

AVRAM M. COOPERMAN

Pancreatic cholera is a rare but spectacular syndrome. Since effective treatment is available, its discussion is included in the present text. It ranks with insulinoma as a devastating illness that is potentially curable.

The association between diarrhea and pancreatic islet cell tumors was first recognized by Gordon and Olivetti[15] in 1947. Stronger evidence linking the conditions was reported by Verner and Morrison[31] in 1958; two patients died of renal and metabolic consequences of hypokalemia, watery diarrhea, and uremia; in both patients benign islet cell tumors were found. The acronym "WDHA," for watery diarrhea, hypokalemia, and achlorhydria, was suggested by Marks and co-workers[19] in 1967. The term pancreatic cholera was suggested by Matsumoto and colleagues,[20] who noted that the profuse diarrhea in these patients was similar to the diarrhea produced by cholera enterotoxin.

Although the entity has generated much discussion and fewer than seventy-five cases have been described, many more patients have been treated or diagnosed but not reported.

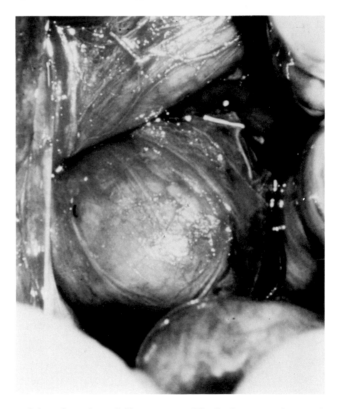

Fig. 10-14. Large right adrenal medullary tumor. The lesion was obscured by the overlying vena cava. (From Cooperman, A. M., et al.: Ann. Surg. In press.)

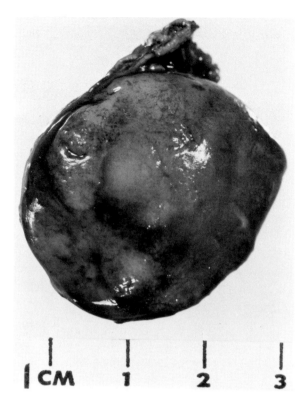

Fig. 10-15. The excised tumor had the histologic appearance of a pheochromocytoma but secreted vasoactive intestinal polypeptide (VIP). Tissue levels of gastrin, calcitonin, cholecystokinin, pancreozymin, prostaglandin, and gastric inhibitory polypeptide (GIP) were normal. Symptomatic cure followed excision of the tumor. (From Cooperman, A. M., et al.: Ann. Surg. In press.)

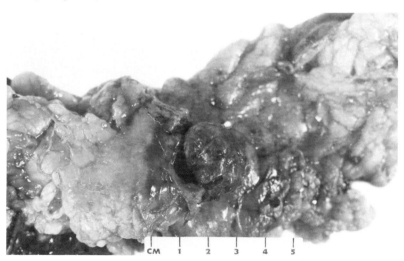

Fig. 10-16. Benign islet cell tumor which caused watery diarrhea. Tissue assay revealed high levels of VIP. All other assays were normal. Cure followed distal pancreatic resection.

A well-recognized fact is that both benign and malignant pancreatic tumors and islet cell hyperplasia (nesidioblastosis) are associated with this syndrome*; but retroperitoneal, pulmonary, and adrenal medullary tumors have also caused watery diarrhea (Figs. 10-14 to 10-16).

Of great interest has been the development of the APUD (amine precursor uptake and decarboxylation) cell concept, particularly as it relates to this and other similar syndromes.[22,32] The term APUD describes common biochemical characteristics shared by these cells and their tumors—APUDomas.[30] These functioning cells produce one or more peptides or hormones and are probably derived from neuroectodermal cells that originate in the neural crest. The APUD cells are totipotential and, in addition to producing a variety of peptides,[7-10] have the ability to migrate to many endodermal and mesodermal tissues, including the foregut, midgut, hindgut, lung, and mediastinum. This clinical spectrum incorporates carcinoid tumors, glucagonomas, gastrinomas, and the watery diarrhea syndrome.[33]

There has been considerable speculation as to what humoral mediator causes the watery diarrhea. In 1968 Zollinger and co-workers[34] suggested that a peptide similar to secretin or a secretin-like substance was the instigating factor. During the past nine years a variety of substances (both hormones and candidate hormones) have been associated or incriminated with this syndrome—including glucagon,[9] vasoactive intestinal polypeptide (VIP),[10,11,14] gastric inhibitory polypeptide (GIP),[10,29] secretin,[27,28,33] and prostaglandin E[17,26]—acting alone or in combination.[28] There has been much evidence (most of it indirect) to support VIP as a causative agent. Of twenty-eight sera assayed from patients with the clinical syndrome, twenty-six had elevated levels of VIP.[25] That multiple peptides may be associated with watery diarrhea was shown by Schmitt and co-workers,[28] who reported a patient with watery diarrhea and a tumor which produced secretin, enteroglucagon, pancreatic glucagon, serotonin, and VIP.

SYMPTOMS

Voluminous watery diarrhea unrelated to diet is the main symptom. It is often abrupt in onset and fulminant in course. The fluid and electrolyte losses, derived mostly from the jejunum,[24] may be so excessive that metabolic acidosis and coma result. One of my patients required more than 400 mEq of KCl in 48 hours to correct hypokalemia prior to surgery.[11]

EVALUATION

Before the watery diarrhea syndrome is suspected, other more common causes of diarrhea must be considered. These include inflammatory

*References 11, 13, 18, 19, 23, 28.

bowel disease, irritable colon, and surreptitious laxative abuse. If findings in all these possibilities prove negative, then stool measurement of bicarbonate and potassium may be helpful. Hypokalemia plus excessive losses of potassium and bicarbonate in the stool are supportive evidence of this syndrome. After the studies, serum should be assayed for all hormones and candidate hormones associated with watery diarrhea. (Only a few laboratories are able to perform these assays, and I have forwarded "blind" specimens to a minimum of three laboratories.) An angiogram is next obtained to outline the pancreas and retroperitoneal vessels in the search for a tumor mass. Angiographic evidence may be positive half the time.

While the serum is being assayed, steroids or indomethacin may be given a trial.[17,23] Relief of watery diarrhea after administration of steroids was noted twenty years ago by Priest and Alexander.[23] The dosage may be minimal, and the relief dramatic. In one of our patients, symptomatic relief and a return of elevated VIP levels to normal occurred within 24 hours after steroid therapy was started. Indomethacin may control watery diarrhea mediated by prostaglandins. Since symptoms can wax and wane, it is important not to attribute relief of diarrhea to a medical program unless the patient is free of symptoms for a prolonged length of time.

If symptoms persist or recur (they usually do), then an operation should be planned. The specific operation will depend on the local findings. When the pancreatic lesion is solitary and benign, excision of the tumor or resection of the gland (depending on its location) has been curative. If a tumor is not found in the pancreas, then a careful exploration of the entire abdomen should be undertaken, including retroperitoneal surfaces, duodenal wall, and adrenal glands.

When a malignant lesion with metastasis is found, decisions regarding appropriate treatment are more difficult. Debulking procedures may initially relieve symptoms by reducing tumor mass but are invariably followed by recurrence. In these isolated circumstances radiotherapy,[26] 5-fluorouracil, and intrahepatic arterial streptozotocin (for liver metastases)[18] have been successful for varying time periods.

On occasion, no tumor is found. For this reason preoperative assay of peptides or hormones may be helpful. If one or more assays show elevated peptides or hormones (in a reliable and sensitive assay), then the surgeon may proceed to do a blind distal pancreatic resection with more justification. It is not known how much pancreas should be resected. The reason to resect pancreas is to look for the presence of islet cell hyperplasia. Thus there is good reason to use this approach.

I prefer resecting pancreas to the left of the superior mensenteric vein. A segment of pancreas is then frozen for histologic examination, and another segment is divided into ten or more portions for peptide hormone assay. If islet cell hyperplasia or elevated hormones are found, further surgery may be necessary to control or prevent recurrence of symptoms. At least eight patients have had islet cell hyperplasia causing this syndrome.[27]

I do not resect more pancreas at an initial operation unless the diagnosis is clear and proved by histologic examination and previous radioimmunoassay. In one interesting case total pancreatectomy was required to control symptoms caused by islet cell hyperplasia after subtotal resection had temporarily controlled diarrhea.[27]

Approximately 40% of tumors are malignant, 40% are benign, and 20% are islet cell hyperplasia. In a few patients no tumor or hyperplasia has been found even at autopsy despite elevated peptide levels. With this situation the course is usually fatal.

Surgical technique

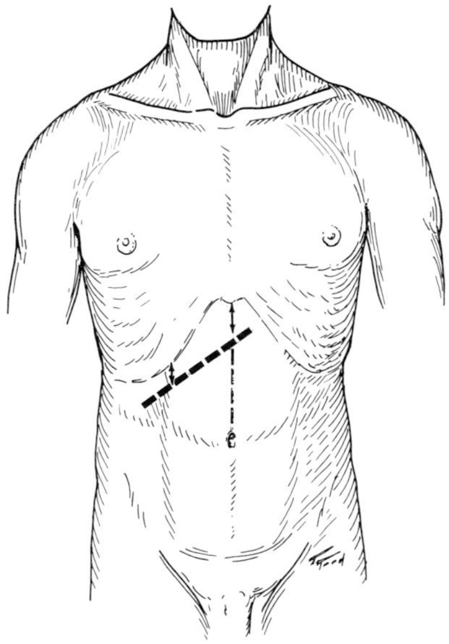

Fig. 10-17. An upper midline incision is preferred, particularly when the tumor has not been localized preoperatively.

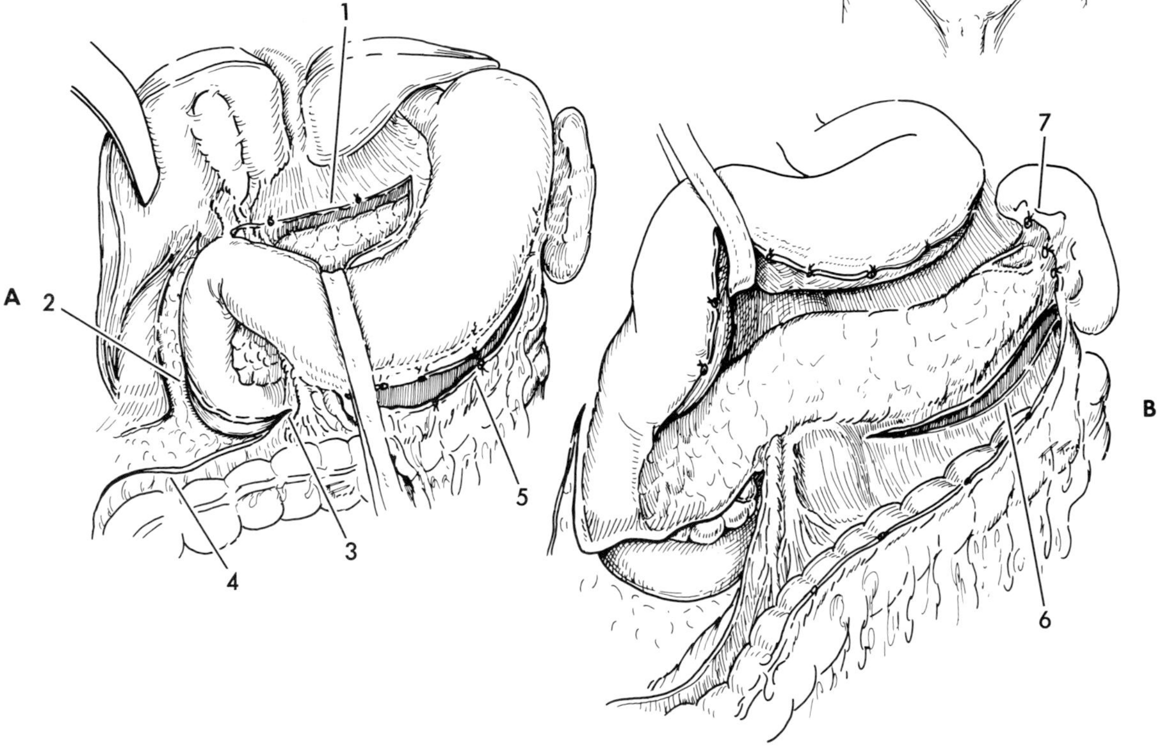

Fig. 10-18. Careful and thorough exploration of the pancreas is done. The seven steps are as outlined in Chapter 1. **A,** A thorough abdominal and pancreatic exploration is done. *1,* The gastrohepatic omentum is incised to expose the body of the pancreas. *2,* The lateral peritoneal reflection is incised over the duodenum and, *3,* is carried to the superior mesenteric vein. *4,* The ascending and right transverse colon may be mobilized in obese patients or if exposure is limited. *5,* The gastrocolic omentum is incised. **B,** *6,* The peritoneum along the inferior border of the pancreas is incised to facilitate bimanual palpation of the body and tail. *7,* If necessary, the spleen and tail of pancreas may be mobilized and delivered anteriorly after the splenorenal ligament has been incised posterolaterally.

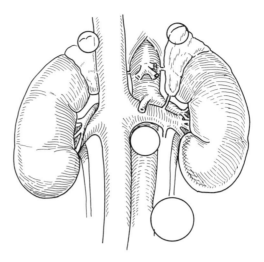

Fig. 10-19. Ectopic locations of tumors should always be considered and sought. Tumors may be in the adrenal glands, the retroperitoneum, or the para-aortic regions.

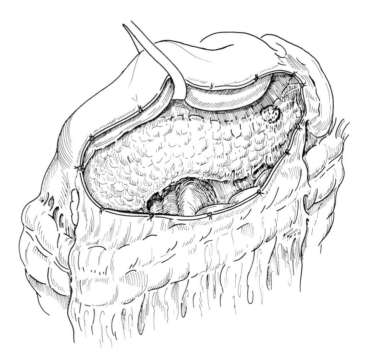

Fig. 10-20. Islet cell tumor in the tail of the pancreas. It produced vasoactive intestinal polypeptide (VIP).

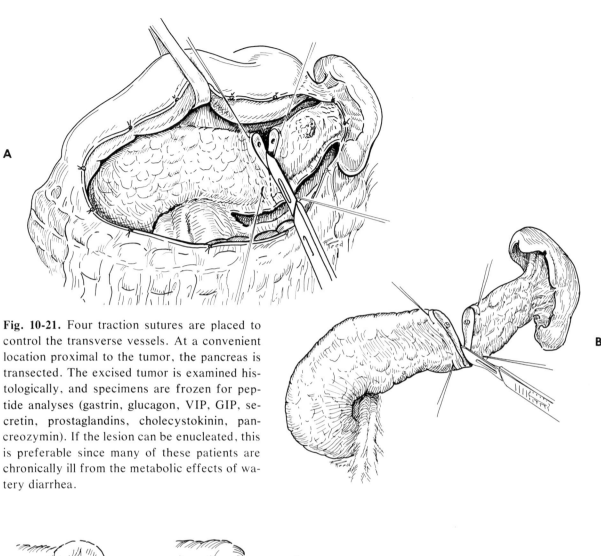

Fig. 10-21. Four traction sutures are placed to control the transverse vessels. At a convenient location proximal to the tumor, the pancreas is transected. The excised tumor is examined histologically, and specimens are frozen for peptide analyses (gastrin, glucagon, VIP, GIP, secretin, prostaglandins, cholecystokinin, pancreozymin). If the lesion can be enucleated, this is preferable since many of these patients are chronically ill from the metabolic effects of watery diarrhea.

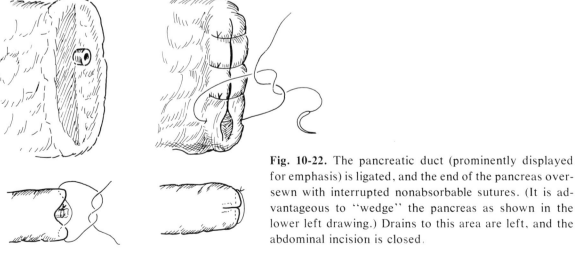

Fig. 10-22. The pancreatic duct (prominently displayed for emphasis) is ligated, and the end of the pancreas oversewn with interrupted nonabsorbable sutures. (It is advantageous to "wedge" the pancreas as shown in the lower left drawing.) Drains to this area are left, and the abdominal incision is closed.

REFERENCES
Insulinomas

1. Alfidi, R. J., Bhyun, D. S., Crile, G., Jr., and Hawk, W.: Arteriography and hypoglycemia, Surg. Gynecol. Obstet. **133:**447, 1971.
2. Campbell, W. R., Graham, R. R., and Robinson, W. L.: Islet cell tumors of the pancreas, Am. J. Med. Sci. **198:**445, 1939.
3. Filipi, C. J., and Higgins, G. A.: Diagnosis and management of insulinoma, Am. J. Surg. **125:**231, 1973.
4. Harris, S.: Hyperinsulinism and dysinsulinism, J.A.M.A. **83:**729, 1924.
5. Nicholls, A. G.: Simple adenoma of the pancreas arising from an island of Langerhans, J. Med. Res. **8:**385, 1902.
6. Whipple, A. O., and Frantz, V. K.: Ademona of islet cells with hyperinsulinism; a review, Ann. Surg. **101:**1299, 1935.
7. Wilder, R. M., Allan, F. N., Power, M. H., and Robertson, H. E.: Carcinoma of the islands of the pancreas; hyperinsulinism and hypoglycemia, J.A.M.A. **89:**348, 1927.

Pancreatic cholera

8. Barbezat, G. O., and Grossman, M. I.: Cholera like diarrhoea induced by glucagon plus gastrin, Lancet **1:**1025, 1971.
9. Barbezat, G. O., and Grossman, M. I.: Intestinal secretion: stimulation by peptides, Gastroenterology **66:**1063, 1974.
10. Bloom, S. R., Polak, J. M., and Pearse, A. G. E.: Vasoactive intestinal peptide and watery diarrhoea syndrome, Lancet **2:**14, 1973.
11. Cooperman, A. M., De Santis, D., Winkelman, E. I., Farmer, R. G., Eversman, J., and Said, S.: The watery diarrhea syndrome, two unpublished cases and further evidence that V.I.P. is a humoral mediator, Ann. Surg. (In press.)
12. Editorial: Hormonally mediated diarrhea, N. Engl. J. Med. **292:**970, 1975.
13. Elias, E., Bloom, S. R., Welbourn, R. B., Kuzio, M., Polak, J. M., Pearse, A. G. E., Booth, C. C., and Brown, J. C.: Pancreatic cholera due to production of gastric inhibitory polypeptide, Lancet **2:**791, 1972.
14. Fausa, O., Fretheim, B., Elgjo, K., Semb, L. S., and Gjone, E.: Intractable watery diarrhoea, hypokalaemia and achlorhydria, associated with non-pancreatic retroperitoneal neurogenous tumour containing vasoactive intestinal peptide (VIP), Scand. J. Gastroenterol. **8:**713, 1973.
15. Gordon, B. S., and Olivetti, R. G.: Carcinoma of the islets of Langerhans: review of the literature and report of two cases, Gastroenterology **9:**409, 1947.
16. Graham, D. Y., Johnson, C. D., Bentlif, P. S., and Kelsey, J. R.: Islet cell carcinoma, pancreatic cholera and vasoactive intestinal peptide, Ann. Intern. Med. **83:**782, 1975.
17. Jaffe, B. M., and Condon, S.: Prostaglandins E and F in endocrine diarrheagenic syndrome, Ann. Surg. **184:**516, 1976.
18. Kahn, C. R., Levy, A. G., Gardner, J. D., Miller, J. V., Gorden, P., and Schein, P. S.: Pancreatic cholera: beneficial effects of treatment with streptozotocin, N. Engl. J. Med. **292:**941, 1975.
19. Marks, I. N., Bank, S., and Louw, J. H.: Islet cell tumor of the pancreas with reversible watery diarrhea and achlorhydria, Gastroenterology **52:**695, 1967.
20. Matsumoto, K. K., Peter, J. B., Schultze, R. G., Hakim, A. A., and Franck, P. T.: Watery diarrhea and hypokalemia associated with pancreatic islet cell adenoma, Gastroenterology **50:**231, 1966.

21. Moore, F. T., Nadler, S. H., Radifeld, D. A., and Zollinger, R. M.: Prolonged remission of diarrhea due to non-beta islet cell tumor of the pancreas by radiotherapy, Am. J. Surg. **115**:854, 1968.

22. Pearse, A. G. E.: Common cytochemical properties of cells producing polypeptide hormones with particular reference to calcitonin and the thyroid C cells, Vet. Rec. **79**:587, 1966.

23. Priest, W. M., and Alexander, M. K.: Islet-cell tumour of the pancreas with peptic ulceration, diarrhoea and hypokalaemia, Lancet **2**:1145, 1957.

24. Rambaud, J. C., Modigliani, R., Matuchansky, C., Bloom, S., Said, S., Pessayre, D., and Bernier, J. J.: Pancreatic cholera: studies on tumoral secretions and pathophysiology of diarrhea, Gastroenterology **69**:110, 1975.

25. Said, S. I., and Faloona, G. R.: Elevated plasma and tissue levels of vasoactive intestinal polypeptide in the watery diarrhea syndrome due to pancreatic, bronchogenic and other tumors, N. Engl. J. Med. **293**:155, 1975.

26. Sandler, M., Karim, S. M. M., and Williams, E. D.: Prostaglandins in amine-peptide-secreting tumours, Lancet **2**:1053, 1968.

27. Sanzenbacher, L. J., Mekhjian, H. S., King, D. R., and Zollinger, R. M.: Studies on the potential role of secretin in the islet cell tumor diarrheogenic syndrome, Ann. Surg. **176**:394, 1972.

28. Schmitt, M. G., Soergel, K. H., Hensley, G. T., and Chey, W. Y.: Watery diarrhea associated with pancreatic islet cell carcinoma, Gastroenterology **69**:206, 1975.

29. Semb, L. S.: Editorial: WDHA-syndrome and gastric secretory inhibitors, Scand. J. Gastroenterology **9**:335, 1974.

30. Szijj, I., Csapó, Z., László, F. A., and Kovács, K.: Medullary cancer of the thyroid gland associated with hypercorticism, Cancer **24**:167, 1969.

31. Verner, J. V., and Morrison, A. B.: Islet cell tumor and a syndrome of refractory watery diarrhea and hypokalemia, Am. J. Med. **25**:374, 1958.

32. Verner, J. V., and Morrison, A. B.: Endocrine pancreatic islet disease with diarrhea. Report of a case due to diffuse hyperplasia of nonbeta islet tissue with a review of 54 additional cases, Arch. Intern. Med. **133**:492, 1974.

33. Welbourn, R. B., Pearse, A. G. E., Polak, J. M., Bloom, S. R., and Joffe, S. N.: The APUD cells of the alimentary tract in health and disease, Med. Clin. North Am. **58**:1359, 1974.

34. Zollinger, R. M., Tompkins, R. K., Amerson, J. R., Endahl, G. L., Kraft, A. R., and Moore, F. T.: Identification of the diarrheogenic hormone associated with non-beta islet cell tumors of the pancreas, Ann. Surg. **168**:502, 1968.

CHAPTER 11

Cystadenoma and cystadenocarcinoma

ROBERT E. HERMANN

Cystic neoplasms of the pancreas continue to be diagnosed relatively infrequently. Approximately 10% of all pancreatic cysts are neoplastic. Less than 400 cases have been reported.

From the several published reviews of cystadenoma and cystadenocarcinoma of the pancreas, it appears that cystadenoma is twice as common as cystadenocarcinoma.[1,2,5,6] Although cystadenoma of the pancreas is a benign tumor, there have been several reports of malignant transformation of these lesions into cystadenocarcinoma.[1,4]

The distinction between a neoplastic cyst of the pancreas and an inflammatory cyst, or pseudocyst, can be made by performing a biopsy of the wall of the cystic lesion. It is also important to open the cyst cavity widely, to debride carefully and gently any tissue extending into the lumen of the cyst, and to include this in the histologic analysis. On one occasion, we performed a biopsy on the wall of a cystadenoma and found fibrous changes consistent with those of a pseudocyst. Only when further tissue was submitted from deeper within the cyst did papillary projections and the other histologic changes of a neoplastic cyst become apparent.

The histologic and histopathologic findings of inflammatory cysts are fibrosis of the wall of the cyst, indicating inflammatory origin. With cystadenoma or cystadenocarcinoma of the pancreas, the tissue lining the cyst is rarely fibrotic. It more frequently consists of flat, cuboidal, or tall columnar epithelial cells. Papillary projections may be recognized either grossly or microscopically in many areas.

Grossly the lesion does not usually occupy the entire pancreas but is a discrete entity, the rest of the pancreas being reasonably normal to appearance and palpation. Although most of the lesion consists of a cyst, areas of solid tissue may be identified.

Neoplastic cysts can vary from small lesions to huge masses filling much of the abdominal cavity. Multiple cysts are usually found though unilocular cysts have also been described. Whenever a multiloculated cyst is encountered at surgery, one should consider a neoplastic cyst. The contents of the cyst may be serous or mucoid material. Occasionally, stromal calcification has been noted in the wall of the cyst. When a cystadenocarcinoma is present, the tumor is usually a slow-growing mass with a low degree of malignancy. Without any areas of obvious distant metastasis or invasion of contiguous structures, it can be difficult to distinguish a cystadenocarcinoma of low-grade malignancy from a benign cystadenoma. For this reason wide local resection of the lesion is the procedure of choice for both types of neoplastic cysts.

CLINICAL FINDINGS

One of the principal clinical characteristics of these lesions is that there is no history of abdominal pain or clinical evidence of pancreatitis. A mass is discovered in the area of the pancreas, with the gradual onset of abdominal discomfort and fullness secondary to the presence of the mass. Pain becomes a clinical symptom gradually in about half of all patients, especially when the cystic lesion becomes large. The pain appears most frequently in the left upper quadrant or epigastrium, with occasional radiation into the back. These lesions tend to be located more in the tail or body and tail of the pancreas than in the head of the gland.

At the time of diagnosis, most patients are between 40 and 60 years of age; however, neoplastic cysts have been reported in teen-agers and in persons who were 70 years or older. There is a striking predominance of cystic neoplasms in women as compared to men, women outnumbering men about 9 to 1 in the incidence of both cystadenoma and cystadenocarcinoma of the pancreas.

DIAGNOSIS

Diagnostic studies may show a mildly elevated amylase level, though most patients will have a normal serum amylase. Plain roentgenograms of the abdomen may disclose the presence of a radiopaque mass. A barium roentgenogram of the upper gastrointestinal tract will usually reveal varying degrees of displacement of the stomach anteriorly, widening of the duodenal C-loop, or effacement of the duodenal mucosa. Barium studies of the colon frequently show downward displacement of the transverse colon. Angiography has been useful in identifying the location of the cystic lesion, its origin in the pancreas, and its relationship to the celiac or superior mesenteric vessels. Frequently, due to stretching of the vessels and the relative avascularity of the lesion, the mass can be identified as a cystic lesion preoperatively.

TREATMENT

Total surgical excision is the treatment of choice for both pancreatic cystadenoma and cystadenocarcinoma. Because of the difficulty in distinguishing between these two lesions and the possibility of malignant change of a benign lesion, every effort should be made to excise the lesion if at all possible.

For lesions in the body or tail of the pancreas, distal pancreatectomy is the treatment of choice. For lesions in the head of the gland, a pancreaticoduodenectomy or Whipple procedure should be performed. For lesions arising in the neck or central area of the pancreas, when firmly adherent to the superior mesenteric vessels, partial or incomplete excision may be possible, leaving a remnant of the cyst wall attached to the vessels.

Simple drainage of the cyst, either internally or by marsupialization to the exterior, should be avoided except as a last resort. Experience with cystogastrostomy, cystojejunostomy, and cystoduodenostomy has shown that the cysts frequently recur with stricturing or stenosis of the opening to the anastomosed loop of gut. Neoplastic tissue may grow into and occlude the anastomotic opening as well.

However, in several reported instances, internal drainage of a cystic lesion has been the only operation possible.[1,3] With such patients significant palliation may be achieved for periods of several years. In some instances repeated operative procedures can be performed to reduce the size of the cyst and rejoin it to an adjacent loop of jejunum by a Roux-en-Y jejunostomy. Becker and co-workers[1] reported one such case; the patient remained healthy ten years after biopsy of a benign cystadenoma of the pancreas and gastrojejunostomy for decompression of a partially obstructed stomach. Long-term survivals have also been reported with patients who underwent marsupialization though the morbidity of a continuing external pancreatic fistula makes internal drainage preferable if at all possible.

Other cystic lesions of the pancreas even more rare have been reported, such as cystic leiomyosarcoma, cystic rhabdomyosarcoma, and cystic islet cell adenoma.[7] Surgical excision of these lesions is the treatment of choice.

Surgical technique

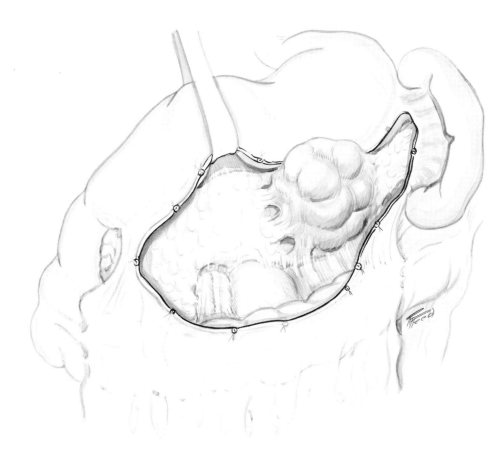

Fig. 11-1. Moderately large cystic tumor of the distal pancreas. The gastrocolic omentum has been opened to explore the pancreas throughout its length. The stomach is retracted superiorly and the colon inferiorly. The pancreas is carefully palpated to determine the extent of the lesion.

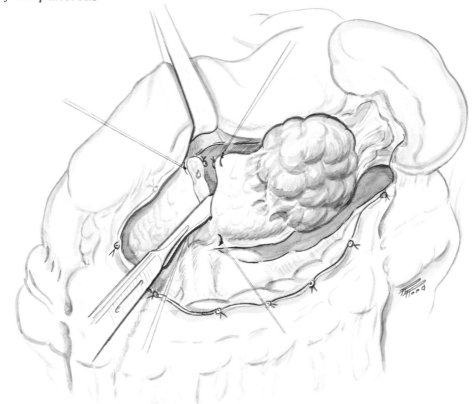

Fig. 11-2. The spleen and distal pancreas have been mobilized anteriorly out of their retroperitoneal position. Blunt dissection behind the pancreas carries the mobilization of the gland to the right to an area of normal pancreas. At this point the splenic artery and vein are isolated and separately ligated. The gland is held with traction sutures of 3-0 silk and divided. The divided pancreatic duct can be seen in the upper central gland. Hemostasis is achieved with fine silk ligatures or by use of the electrocautery on small intrapancreatic vessels.

Fig. 11-3. Management of the divided pancreas. Hemostasis of fine blood vessels has been achieved. The pancreatic duct is separately isolated and ligated (or suture ligated) with 3-0 silk. The divided end of the gland (which is beveled to permit its closure) is then oversewn with interrupted sutures (or mattress sutures) of 3-0 silk. A Penrose drain or sump suction drain is usually left for several days after surgery.

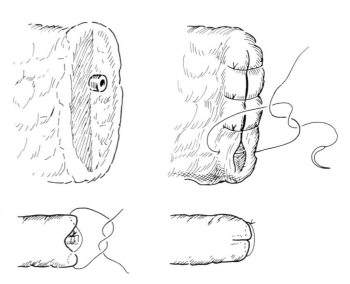

REFERENCES

1. Becker, W. F., Welsh, R. A., and Pratt, H. S.: Cystadenoma and cystadenocarcinoma of the pancreas, Ann. Surg. **161:**845, 1965.
2. Didolkar, M. S., Malhotra, Y., Holyoke, E. D., and Elias, E. G.: Cystadenoma of the pancreas, Surg. Gynecol. Obstet. **140:**925, 1975.
3. Piper, C. E., Jr., ReMine, W. H., and Priestley, J. T.: Pancreatic cystadenomata; report of 20 cases, J.A.M.A. **180:**648, 1962.
4. Probstein, J. G., and Blumenthal, H. T.: Progressive malignant degeneration of a cystadenoma of the pancreas, Arch. Surg. **81:**683, 1960.
5. Sawyer, R. B., Sawyer, K. C., and Spencer, J. R.: Proliferative cysts of the pancreas, Am. J. Surg. **116:**763, 1968.
6. Warren, K. W., Athanassiades, S., Frederick, P., and Kune, G. A.: Surgical treatment of pancreatic cysts; review of 183 cases, Ann. Surg. **163:**886, 1966.
7. Winston, J. H., Jr.: Malignant islet cell adenoma in a pancreatic cyst; report of a case, J. Natl. Med. Assoc. **57:**203-204, 1965.

CHAPTER 12

Benign tumors of the ampulla of Vater

AVRAM M. COOPERMAN

Benign tumors of the ampulla of Vater are uncommon lesions that may be asymptomatic and discovered at autopsy or symptomatic and presenting a clinical picture of common bile duct or pancreatic duct obstruction.*

The most common of these benign lesions are usually polypoid villous tumors that range in size from 4 mm to 7 cm.[2,19] They have been designated as papillomas, villous adenomas, or polypoid tumors† (Figs. 12-1 and 12-2). Other benign lesions include lymphangiomas, carcinoid tumors, leiomyomas, lipomas, neurogenic tumors, and hemangiomas.‡

The incidence of benign ampullary lesions in autopsy and clinical studies is 0.04% to 0.12%[2]; but it is difficult to determine the true incidence of these lesions because some have been included and classified with duodenal, bile duct, and terminal pancreatic duct tumors. An estimated ninety to 100 cases have been reported in the world literature, and forty-five symptomatic cases have been summarized in the English literature.[26]

SYMPTOMS AND DIAGNOSIS

Obstructive symptoms caused by ampullary tumors are intermittent and simulate cholecystitis, choledocholithiasis,[19,26] or pancreatitis.[21] Duodenal obstruction (25% of cases) or bleeding secondary to tumor ulcera-

My appreciation to Steven Sobol, M.D., who gathered the reference material for this chapter.
*References 1, 3, 4, 6, 8, 11, 18, 20, 22, 23.
†References 1, 2, 4, 6, 8, 11, 18, 19, 20.
‡References 3, 5, 7, 9, 10, 12, 13, 14, 16, 25.

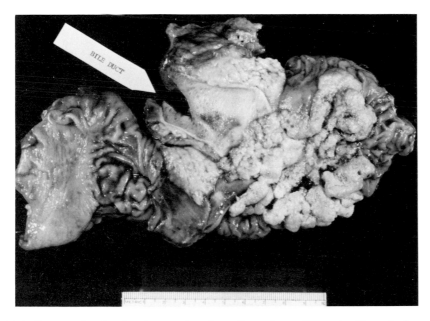

Fig. 12-1. Pancreaticoduodenal resection done for a large (10 cm) villous lesion of the ampulla of Vater. The lesion was benign and the patient survives twenty years later.

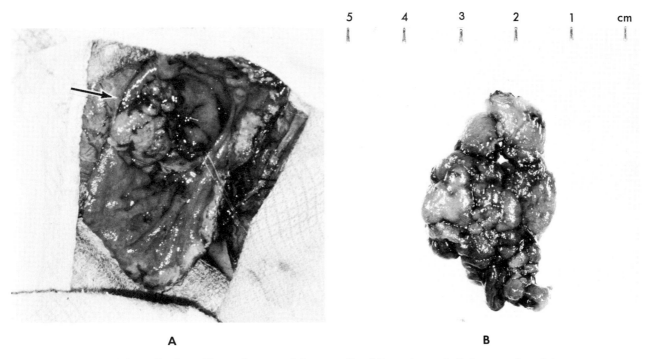

Fig. 12-2. A, Benign villous adenoma of the ampulla of Vater (arrow). Submucosal excision was successfully performed. **B,** The excised lesion. (From Sobol, S., and Cooperman, A.: Gastroenterology. In press.)

tion is less common.[15] Jaundice has been a presenting symptom in 80% of the reported cases.[26]

The diagnosis is often difficult to establish, usually because the entity is not thought of preoperatively. Oral cholecystography and intravenous cholangiography may show only a dilated common bile duct. Associated gallstones are noted in 13% to 20% of cases.[24,26] Widespread use of endoscopy and more frequent use of operative choledochoscopy in symptomatic patients with normal gallbladder studies may allow this diagnosis to be made more often preoperatively or at surgery in patients explored for biliary disease.

In patients who are explored for biliary disease and in whom operative cholangiograms are normal, distal duct obstruction must be excluded. Even if no tumor is palpated through the duodenum at the ampulla, the diagnosis cannot be excluded since the lesion may be small. At times open duodenotomy and visualization of the ampulla are required to establish the diagnosis.

TREATMENT

Treatment for benign ampullary tumors varies but most often involves submucosal resection of the ampulla.[9] Of forty-five operations reported in the American literature, this has been sufficient treatment in most.[26] Because the pancreatic and bile ducts will be transected by submucosal transection of the ampulla, some surgeons have advocated reimplanting the ducts in the duodenal wall.[17] When the ducts have been dilated from chronic obstruction, this may be unnecessary.

When the ducts are normal in size, sphincteroplasty may be done. There is little objective evidence to help make the decision. When the ducts are of normal size, I prefer to perform sphincteroplasty on the common bile duct and insert a small nonobstructing catheter into the orifice of the pancreatic duct or do a short sphincteroplasty on the pancreatic duct.[26] A suitable alternative may be to do a cholecystojejunostomy in case a stricture of the distal duct develops.

When the tumor has in situ malignant changes, submucosal resection is probably still adequate treatment. The incidence of malignant changes (in situ and invasive) in villous tumors of the ampulla varies from 5% to 35%.[9,26]

For invasive cancers the treatment should be the same as for invasive papillary cancers, either pancreaticoduodenal resection or biliary enteric bypass depending on the general condition of the patient and the local findings.

Surgical technique

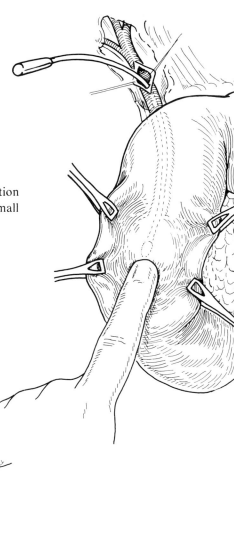

Fig. 12-3. The ampulla may be located by digital palpation of the descending duodenum or by passage of a small probe into the common bile duct.

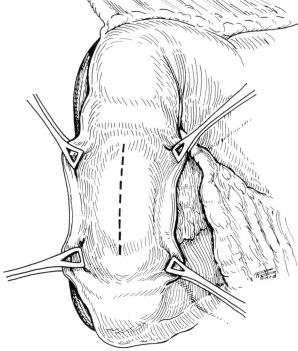

Fig. 12-4. A longitudinal incision is made over the ampullary area.

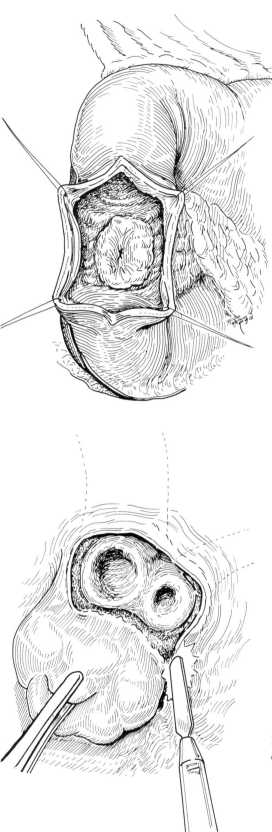

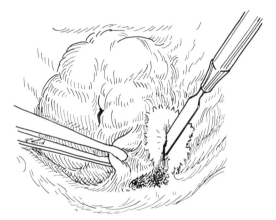

Fig. 12-5. Polypoid ampullary tumor. Four traction sutures or small right-angle retractors facilitate exposure. A Kocher maneuver will deliver the duodenum anteriorly.

Fig. 12-6. A cautery unit (our preference) facilitates hemostasis and submucosal removal of the lesion.

Fig. 12-7. As the tumor is excised, the orifices of the common bile duct and pancreatic duct are visualized.

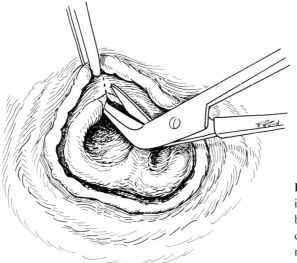

Fig. 12-8. A sphincteroplasty in the common bile duct is made by excision of a wedge of anterior common bile duct wall. This procedure may prevent a distal duct stricture from developing, but the need for it is not known.

Fig. 12-9. It is even less clear how to deal with the pancreatic duct. If the duct is dilated, nothing is done. If the duct is of normal size, a short sphincteroplasty is performed or a small nonobstructing catheter is inserted, with the expectation that the catheter will pass spontaneously in weeks or months.

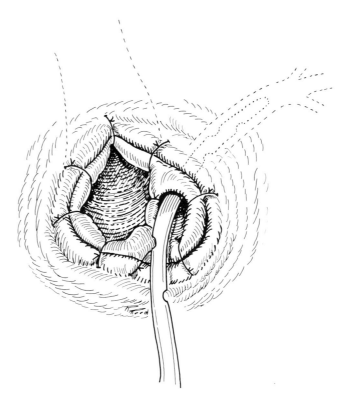

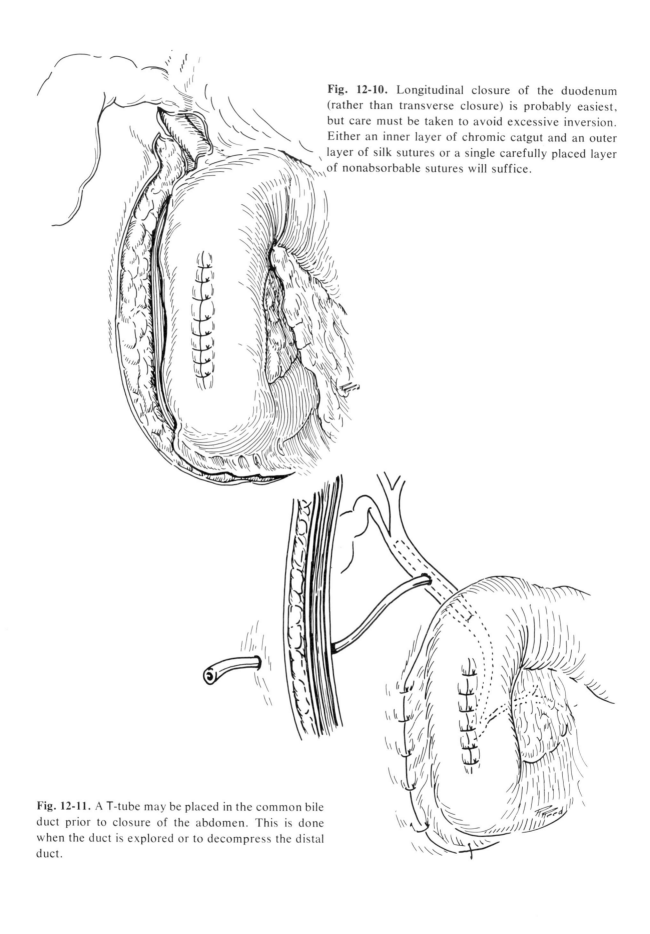

Fig. 12-10. Longitudinal closure of the duodenum (rather than transverse closure) is probably easiest, but care must be taken to avoid excessive inversion. Either an inner layer of chromic catgut and an outer layer of silk sutures or a single carefully placed layer of nonabsorbable sutures will suffice.

Fig. 12-11. A T-tube may be placed in the common bile duct prior to closure of the abdomen. This is done when the duct is explored or to decompress the distal duct.

REFERENCES

1. Anderson, M. C., and Gregor, W. H.: Papilloma of the ampulla of Vater, Am. J. Surg. **102:**865, 1961.
2. Baggenstoss, A. M.: Major duodenal papilla: variations of pathologic interest and lesions of mucosa, Proc. Staff Meet. Mayo Clin. **13:**29, 1938.
3. Baker, H. L., and Caldwell, D. W.: Lesions of the ampulla of Vater, Surgery **21:**523, 1947.
4. Barbanera, M., and Destefani, A.: A case of giant papilloma of the ampulla of Vater, Rass. Arch. Chir. **10:**9, 1972.
5. Barber, K. W., Jr., ReMine, W. H., Harrison, E. G., Jr., and Priestley, J. T.: Benign neoplasms of extrahepatic bile ducts, including papilla of Vater, Arch. Surg. **81:**479, 1960.
6. Bremer, E. H., Battaile, W. G., and Bulle, P. H.: Villous tumors of the upper gastrointestinal tract, Am. J. Gastroenterol. **50:**135, 1968.
7. Brombart, M., Henry, C., and Delcourt, R.: Sur quelques cas de tumeurs bénignes de l'ampoule de Vater, Acta Gastroenterol. Belg. **21:**230, 1958.
8. Cattell, R. B., Braasch, J. W., and Kahn, F.: Polypoid epithelial tumors of the bile ducts, N. Engl. J. Med. **266:**57, 1962.
9. Cattell, R. B., and Pyrtek, L. J.: Premalignant lesions of the ampulla of Vater, Surg. Gynecol. Obstet. **90:**21, 1950.
10. Chatelin, C. L., and Denjoy, R.: Les tumeurs bénignes de la papille de Vater; à propos de 5 observations, J. Chir. **88:**45, 1964.
11. Christopher, F.: Adenoma of the ampulla of Vater, Surg. Gynecol. Obstet. **56:**202, 1933.
12. Curry, B., and Gray, N.: Visceral neurofibromatosis. An unusual cause of obstructive jaundice, Br. J. Surg. **59:**494, 1972.
13. D'Alonzo, U.: Carcinoid of the ampulla of Vater, Opsed. Ital. Chir. **19:**261, 1968.
14. Denjoy, R.: Les tumeurs bénignes de la papille de Vater, J. Chir. **95:**211, 1968.
15. Goldstein, H. S., and Daviglus, G. F.: Benign adenomatous polyp of the papilla of Vater with partial obstruction, Ann. Surg. **160:**844, 1964.
16. Gröbl, W., and Pohl, W.: Ueber die Tumoren der äusseren Gallenwege (Erfahrungen an Hand eines Krankengutes von 206 Fällen), Beitr. Klin. Chir. **173:**215, 1942.
17. Kavlie, H., Dillard, D. H., and White, T. T.: Duodenectomy with reimplantation of the papilla into the jejunum as a treatment for benign duodenal lesions, Surgery **73:**230, 1973.
18. Meltzer, A. D., Ostrum, B. J., and Isard, H. J.: Villous tumors of the stomach and duodenum, Radiology **87:**511, 1966.
19. Mir-Madjlessi, S. H., Farmer, R. G., and Hawk, W.: Villous tumors of the duodenum and jejunum, Am. J. Dig. Dis. **18:**467, 1973.
20. Oh, C., and Jemerin, E. E.: Benign adenomatous polyps of the papilla of Vater, Surgery **57:**495, 1965.
21. Ohmori, K., Kiroshita, H., Shiraha, Y., and Satake, K.: Pancreatic duct obstruction by a benign polypoid adenoma of the ampulla of Vater, Am. J. Surg. **132:**662, 1976.
22. Poilleux, J.: Les tumeurs bénignes de la région Vatérienne, Med. Chir. Dig. **4:**25, 1975.
23. Ring, E. J., Ferrucci, J. T., Eaton, S. B., Jr., and Clements, J. L.: Villous adenomas of the duodenum, Radiology **104:**45, 1972.
24. Schulten, M. F., Oyasu, R., and Beal, J. M.: Villous adenomas of the duodenum. Case report and review of the literature, Am. J. Surg. **132:**90, 1976.
25. Shapiro, P. F., and Lifvendahl, R. A.: Tumors of the extrahepatic bile-ducts, Ann. Surg. **94:**61, 1931.
26. Sobol, S., and Cooperman, A.: Benign polypoid ampullary tumor; a case report and review of the world literature, Gastroenterology. (In press.)

CHAPTER 13

Annular pancreas

AVRAM M. COOPERMAN

Annular pancreas is an uncommon cause of duodenal obstruction. Although most often presenting as symptomatic duodenal obstruction in infancy and childhood, annular pancreas may not become manifest until later life. In recent reviews more than 250 cases were reported in adults,[3,7] most of them since 1952. Undoubtedly many more cases have been treated but not reported or have been included in reports of other benign obstructing duodenal lesions (webs, ulcers, bands).

Several theories have been proposed to explain the genesis of this lesion. A popular theory is that the annulus is caused by fixation of a portion of the ventral pancreas as it migrates to the right and posterior to the duodenum where it fuses with the dorsal segment.[1] Because it remains encircled about the duodenum, the dorsal portion may develop symptomatic obstruction. Occasionally only a posterior segment of the annulus remains fixed. This is the incomplete form. Why this happens is unclear. Possible explanations include lack of fusion, failure of rotation, and persistence of a ventral segment.

The commonest presenting complaint relates to duodenal obstruction. Occasionally obstructive jaundice or pancreatitis is an accompanying symptom. Congenital anomalies of the intestinal tract are uncommon in adults.[8] Associated duodenal ulcer (postulated to be due to stasis or lack of acid neutralization by obstructed alkaline secretions) has been incriminated in up to 43% of adult cases.[3] In one series the presence of duodenal ulcer correlated with the presence of long-standing symptoms from the annulus.[3]

The diagnosis is suggested by barium roentgenographic studies which show a smooth symmetric hourglass annular filling defect in the second portion of the duodenum, dilatation of the proximal duodenum, and occasionally reverse peristalsis in the duodenum proximal to the annulus.[4,5,7]

TREATMENT (SURGERY)

At surgery the diagnosis may be difficult, particularly if a coexisting proximal duodenal ulcer is present or if the annular segment lies posteriorly and cannot be visualized. To establish the diagnosis, the descending duodenum must be mobilized to the vena cava by incising the lateral peritoneum of the duodenum.

There are at least two surgical options in treating annular pancreas in adults: (1) bypass of the obstructed area and (2) resection of the annulus. Reemstma[6] reviewed 101 patients treated surgically by both procedures. Although the mortality rate was similar after each, the incidence of complications after division of the annulus was 55% as compared to 10% after bypass.

There are two theoretical objections to annular division: (1) a major pancreatic duct coursing through the annular segment may be unavoidably divided and (2) the duodenum may not expand beneath the division of annulus because its normal elasticity is irreversibly fibrosed[6,8] or the annular segment has become enmeshed in the duodenal wall.[1]

The most popular operation is a bypass procedure, preferably a duodenoduodenostomy or, failing that, a duodenojejunostomy. This anastomosis will function by peristalsis and hydrostatic pressure. Although gastrojejunostomy has been utilized, it is less desirable because there are theoretical and practical objections to its use: the high likelihood that the stomach will empty first through the pylorus and then reflux back into the stomach and jejunum, a higher incidence of biliary or alkaline gastritis following gastrojejunostomy, and a tendency to develop marginal ulcers. These complications have been reported.

If an associated duodenal ulcer is present, a vagotomy and resection or vagotomy and drainage procedure may also be required. (In this instance gastrojejunostomy is a good choice.) One wonders whether relief of the duodenal obstruction alone might cure the ulcer (if it is caused by stasis). This thought is not likely to be answered by clinical studies, and the recommended treatment will continue to be an operation that includes relief of the duodenal obstruction plus correction of the ulcer.

I prefer vagotomy plus gastrojejunostomy or highly selective vagotomy plus duodenojejunostomy. With the increasing use of highly selective vagotomy, this may be an ideal condition for the operation, provided the long-term results are satisfactory.

When coexisting biliary disease is present, careful attention to common duct anatomy is necessary. Cholangiography to detail the gallbladder and bile duct will guide accurate treatment and occasionally will outline the pancreatic duct in the annular segment as well.[7,9]

The results of these operations are uniformly successful. Whether this is because follow-up is not stated, or mechanical relief of the obstruction ensures a satisfactory result is not totally clear. I suspect the latter is correct both from a small personal experience and from Lloyd Jones' review in which eight patients were well more than five years after surgical correction.[3]

Surgical technique

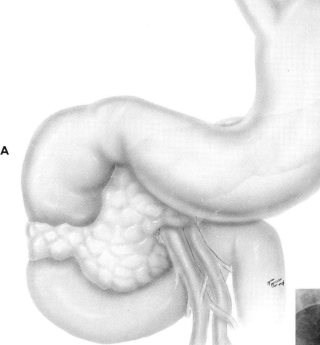

A

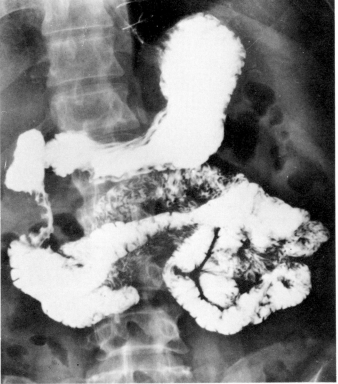

B

Fig. 13-1. A, Obstruction of the middle descending duodenum by a completely annular pancreas. **B,** Annular pancreas in the adult. A long smooth obstruction of the descending duodenum (annular segment) with proximal dilatation of the duodenum is seen.

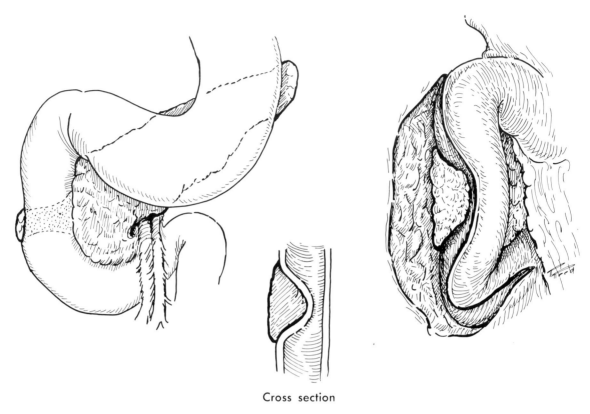

Cross section

Fig. 13-2. Incomplete form of annular pancreas. It is necessary to mobilize the descending duodenum so visual and manual inspection can be done.

Fig. 13-3. Because the main pancreatic duct may course through the annular segment, the area is bypassed and not resected. To preserve the integrity of the pylorus and prevent reflux, the bypass used is a side-to-side duodenoduodenostomy. If the duodenum cannot be mobilized, a loop of jejunum may be brought up through the mesocolon and a duodenojejunostomy used. A posterior row of interrupted nonabsorbable 4-0 silk sutures is first placed and tied.

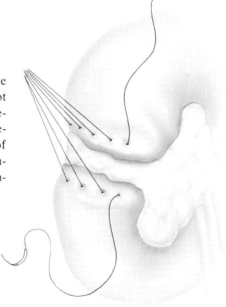

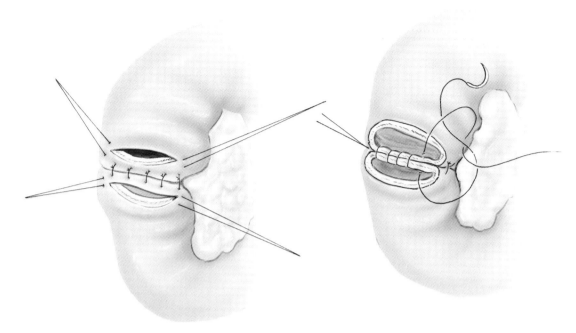

Fig. 13-4. The sutures are cut after the lumen is opened on both sides of the obstruction. A posterior row of running or interrupted 4-0 chromic catgut is placed and continued as a simple running inverting stitch anteriorly.

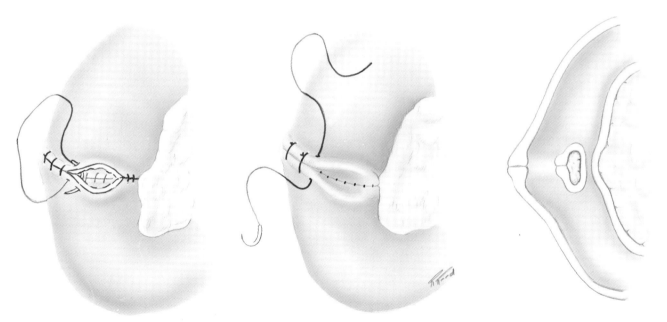

Fig. 13-5. An outer anterior seromuscular layer of 3-0 silk sutures is placed and tied. The completed anastomosis is viewed in cross section showing the intact annular segment. Single-layer anterior closure may also be utilized.

REFERENCES

1. Hyden, W. H.: The true nature of annular pancreas, Ann. Surg. **157:**71, 1963.
2. Lecco, T. M. Quoted by Howard, J. M.: Annular pancreas, Surg. Gynecol. Obstet. **50:**533, 1930.
3. Lloyd-Jones, W., Mountain, J. C., and Warren, K. W.: Annular pancreas in the adult, Ann. Surg. **176:**163, 1972.
4. Mast, W. H., Telle, L. D., and Turek, R. O.: Annular pancreas: errors in diagnosis and treatment of eight cases, Am. J. Surg. **94:**80, 1957.
5. Poppel, M. H., and Marshak, R. H.: Roentgen diagnosis of pancreatic disease, Am. J. Roentgenol. Radium Ther. Nucl. Med. **170:**163, 1972.
6. Reemtsma, K.: Embryology and congenital anomalies of the pancreas. In Howard, J. M., and Jordan, G. L., editors: Surgical disease of the pancreas, Philadelphia, 1960, J. B. Lippincott Co.
7. Seliger, G., and Goldman, A.: Symptomatic annular pancreas in a 75-year old man, Am. J. Gastroenterol. **60:**185, 1973.
8. Stofer, B. E.: Annular pancreas: a tabulation of the recent literature and report of a case, Am. J. Med. Sci. **207:**430, 1944.
9. Whelan, T. J., Jr., and Hamilton, G. B.: Annular pancreas, Ann. Surg. **146:**252, 1957.

INDEX